CMSRN

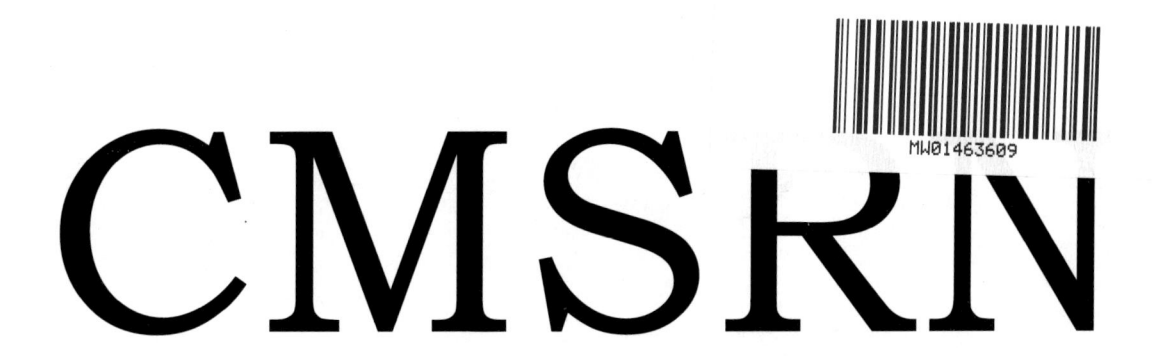

EXAM PREP
2024-2025

Achieve Excellence in Med Surg Certification!
Tests | Q&A | Extra Content

Robert Cliven

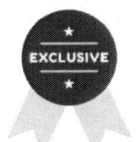

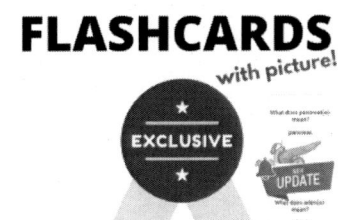

© Copyright **2023** by **Robert Cliven** - All rights reserved.

The following Book is reproduced below to provide information that is as accurate and reliable as possible. Regardless, purchasing this Book can be seen as consent to the fact that both the publisher and the author of this book are in no way experts on the topics discussed within and that any recommendations or suggestions that are made herein are for entertainment purposes only. Professionals should be consulted as needed prior to undertaking any of the action endorsed herein.

This declaration is deemed fair and valid by both the American Bar Association and the Committee of Publishers Association and is legally binding throughout the United States. Furthermore, the transmission, duplication, or reproduction of any of the following work including specific information will be considered an illegal act irrespective of if it is done electronically or in print. This extends to creating a secondary or tertiary copy of the work or a recorded copy and is only allowed with the express written consent from the Publisher. All additional right reserved..

Additionally, the information in the following pages is intended only for informational purposes and should thus be thought of as universal. As befitting its nature, it is presented without assurance regarding its prolonged validity or interim quality. Trademarks that are mentioned are done without written consent and can in no way be considered an endorsement from the trademark holder.

EXLUSIVE EXTRA CONTENTS FOR YOU IN THE LAST CHAPTER!

I have recently decided to give **gifts** to all our readers. Yes, I want to provide you with the assistance that will help you with your study you will receive:

- *Audiobook*
- eBook: "*Medical Terminology for Health Careers*"
- **+600 flashcards with pictures** of "*Medical Terms*"
- Practical *Case Studies*
- *Digital version of this book*

Extra content for you
CASE STUDIES

Extra content for you
FLASHCARDS with picture!

Extra content for you
AUDIOBOOK

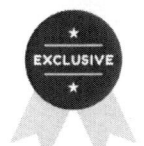

You can track your progress and conveniently and interactively memorize the most important terms and concepts! Learn with printable flashcards or interactive flashcards on your device with **Anki APP or AnkiDroid!**

TABLE OF CONTENTS

INTRODUCTION 11

CARDIOVASCULAR NURSING 13

Heart and Vascular Diseases 14
- Coronary artery disease (CAD) 14
- Myocardial Infarction (MI) 14
- Congestive Heart Failure (CHF) 14
- Arrhythmias 14
- Hypertension 14
- Peripheral Artery Disease (PAD) 14

Interventions and Treatments 15
- Pharmacologic Therapies 15
- Surgical Interventions 15
- Lifestyle Modifications 15
  - Rehabilitation 16
  - Heart Valve Surgery 16
  - Heart Transplant 16
  - Ventricular Assist Devices (VADs) 16
  - Medication Adherence 16
  - Patient and Family Education 16
  - End-of-Life Care 16
  - Continuing Research and Evidence-Based Practice 16

PULMONARY NURSING 17

Respiratory Disorders 18
- Chronic Obstructive Pulmonary Disease (COPD) 18
- Asthma 18
- Pneumonia 18
- Tuberculosis (TB) 18
- Lung Cancer 18
- Pulmonary Embolism (PE) 18
- Pulmonary Hypertension 19
- Cystic Fibrosis (CF) 19
- Idiopathic Pulmonary Fibrosis (IPF) 19
- Sarcoidosis 19
- Sleep Apnea 19
- Pleural Effusion 19
- Pneumothorax 20

Interventions and Treatments 20
- Pharmacologic Treatments 20
- Oxygen Therapy 20
- Breathing Techniques 20
- Pulmonary Rehabilitation 20
- Surgical Interventions 20
- Patient Education 21
- Palliative Care 21
- Nebulizer Treatments 21
- Chest Physiotherapy 21
- Positive Pressure Ventilation 21

Tracheostomy Care 21
Smoking Cessation Programs 21
Vaccinations 22
End-of-Life Care 22

GASTROINTESTINAL NURSING 23

Digestive Disorders 23
Gastroesophageal Reflux Disease (GERD) 23
Peptic Ulcer Disease (PUD) 24
Gastritis 24
Inflammatory Bowel Disease (IBD) 24
Irritable Bowel Syndrome (IBS) 24
Gallstones 24
Hepatitis 24
Cirrhosis 24
Pancreatitis 24
Colorectal Cancer 25
Diverticular Disease 25
Celiac Disease 25
Gastroenteritis 25
Anal Fissures 25
Hemorrhoids 25

Interventions and Treatments 26
Pharmacological Interventions 26
Surgical Interventions 26
Dietary Interventions 26
Lifestyle Modifications 26
Therapeutic Procedures 26
Palliative Care 27
Patient Education 27

RENAL AND URINARY NURSING 29

Kidney and Urinary Tract Disorders 30
Acute Kidney Injury (AKI) 30
Chronic Kidney Disease (CKD) 30
Urinary Tract Infections (UTIs) 30
Kidney Stones 30
Glomerulonephritis 30
Polycystic Kidney Disease (PKD) 30
Renal Artery Stenosis 30
Bladder Disorders 31
Nephrotic Syndrome 31
Hydronephrosis 31
Urinary Incontinence 31
Renal Cell Carcinoma (R.C.C.) 31
Vesicoureteral Reflux (VUR) 31
Pyelonephritis 31
Interstitial Cystitis (IC) 31
Prostatitis 31

Interventions and Treatments 32
Treatment Strategies for Acute Kidney Injury (AKI) 32
Management of Chronic Kidney Disease (CKD) 32
Approaches for Polycystic Kidney Disease (PKD) 32
Managing Glomerulonephritis 32
Interventions for Kidney Stones 32
Dealing with Nephrotic Syndrome 32

Hydronephrosis Management 33
Interventions for Renal Cell Carcinoma (RCC) 33
Vesicoureteral Reflux (V.U.R.) Treatment 33
Pyelonephritis Interventions 33
Interstitial Cystitis (IC.) Management 33
Prostatitis Treatment 33

NEUROLOGICAL NURSING 35

Neurological Disorders 36
Stroke 36
Epilepsy 36
Neurodegenerative diseases 36
Multiple sclerosis (MS) 36
Amyotrophic lateral sclerosis (ALS) 36
Guillain-Barre 36
Traumatic brain injury (TBI) 37

Interventions and Treatments 37
Stroke Intervention and Treatment 37
Epilepsy Management 37
Neurodegenerative Disease Management 37
Multiple Sclerosis (MS.) Treatment 37
Amyotrophic Lateral Sclerosis (ALS.) Management 37
Guillain-Barre Syndrome Treatment 38
Traumatic Brain Injury (TBI.) Management 38
Migraine and Headache Management 38
Spinal Cord Injury Treatment 38
Peripheral Neuropathy Management 38
Neuromuscular Disorders Treatment 38
Sleep Disorders Management 38

MUSCULOSKELETAL NURSING 39

Musculoskeletal Disorders 39
Fractures 39
Sprains and Strains 40
Osteoarthritis (OA) 40
Rheumatoid Arthritis (RA) 40
Osteoporosis 40
Musculoskeletal Back Pain 40
Gout 40
Fibromyalgia 40
Systemic Lupus Erythematosus (SLE) 41
Tendinitis 41
Carpal Tunnel Syndrome 41

Interventions and Treatments 41
Pain Management 41
Physical Therapy and Rehabilitation 41
Orthotic Devices 41
Surgical Interventions 42
Lifestyle Modifications 42
Complementary Therapies 42
Medication Management 42
Patient Education 42
Psychosocial Support 42
Intravenous and Subcutaneous Therapies 42
Occupational Therapy 43
Use of Heat and Cold 43

Assistive Devices 43
Joint Injections 43
Advanced Surgical Interventions 43
Comprehensive Pain Management 43
Support Groups and Counseling 43
Preventive Care and Screening 43

PRACTICE TEST 44

Cardiovascular Nursing 44

Pulmonary Nursing 47

Gastrointestinal Nursing 49

Renal and Urinary Nursing 51

Neurological Nursing 53

Musculoskeletal Nursing 55

Endocrine Nursing 57

Hematological and Immunological Nursing 59

ANSWER KEY 63

Cardiovascular Nursing 63

Pulmonary Nursing 64

Gastrointestinal Nursing 65

Renal and Urinary Nursing 66

Neurological Nursing 67

Musculoskeletal Nursing 68

Endocrine Nursing 69

Hematological and Immunological Nursing 70

FAQS PART 1 71

FAQS PART 2 77

CONCLUSION 87

SPECIAL EXTRA CONTENT 89

INTRODUCTION

Welcome to the first step of your journey toward becoming a Certified Medical-Surgical Registered Nurse (CMSRN). This distinction, recognized across the healthcare industry, represents a level of commitment and expertise that sets you apart in medical-surgical nursing.

The CMSRN examination, developed by the Medical-Surgical Nursing Certification Board (MSNCB), assesses your understanding of various clinical topics, patient populations, and settings within the med-surg specialty. The exam has been meticulously structured to align with the practical, everyday experiences of nurses working in medical-surgical settings.

The examination consists of 150 multiple-choice questions, including 25 pretest items that do not count toward your final score. These questions delve into a broad spectrum of topics, from acute care and health promotion to pain management and end-of-life care. The goal is to evaluate your ability to provide optimal patient care, promote health, and adapt to the ever-changing environments typical of a medical-surgical nursing setting.

The CMSRN is not just another certificate; it's a testimony to your dedication, showcasing your competency and command over the intricacies of medical-surgical nursing. Moreover, earning this certification brings numerous professional benefits. Besides fostering your career progression, it bolsters your confidence, sharpens your critical thinking, and enhances your credibility among peers and patients.

Passing the CMSRN exam requires diligence, effective study techniques, and a comprehensive understanding of the field. Don't worry if you feel overwhelmed; this book is designed to guide you step-by-step through the entire process. With practice questions, detailed explanations, and a focused review of key concepts, this study guide aims to provide you with the knowledge and confidence to ace the CMSRN exam.

Remember, every healthcare journey is unique, just as every patient. As you prepare for the CMSRN exam, consider it a means to empower yourself, uplift your nursing practice, and ultimately provide exceptional care to those who need it most.

Together, we will explore the world of medical-surgical nursing, delve deep into its realms, and work towards achieving your CMSRN certification. Let's get started on this exciting journey!

As we embark on this journey together, it's vital to understand the CMSRN exam's structure and content clearly. This comprehensive assessment is a powerful tool for measuring your medical-surgical nursing skills, knowledge, and abilities.

The exam's content revolves around seven domains, reflecting critical aspects of medical-surgical nursing practice. These are as follows.

- Musculoskeletal and Neurological
- Gastrointestinal, Genitourinary, and Renal
- Cardiovascular and Pulmonary
- Endocrine, Hematological, Immunological, and Integumentary
- Eye, Ear, Nose, and Throat; and Reproductive
- Professional Practice
- Acute Care/Subacute/Chronic Illness

Each domain contributes to a different percentage of the total exam questions, and this guide will provide a comprehensive review of all these domains. Understanding the intricacies of each one will equip you with the necessary tools to tackle the exam and provide exceptional patient care confidently.

The CMSRN exam uses a computer-based testing (CBT) format, allowing you to take the exam at many nationwide testing centers. You'll receive instant feedback about your pass/fail status, minimizing the anxious wait.

Taking the CMSRN exam demonstrates your commitment to improving patient outcomes and pursuing professional growth. It requires intensive preparation and a solid grounding in medical-surgical nursing concepts and practices.

Yet, despite its complexity, this exam is manageable. With diligent preparation, steadfast dedication, and this comprehensive guide, you'll be well on your way to earning the coveted CMSRN credential and enhancing the quality of care you deliver.

CARDIOVASCULAR NURSING

Diving into the crux of medical-surgical nursing, we start with an essential domain: Cardiovascular Nursing. Understanding the heart and the vascular system is more than memorizing the anatomy. It's about delving into how these systems function, what can disrupt their harmony, and, most importantly, how we can help restore that equilibrium as nurses.

Cardiovascular nursing involves caring for patients suffering from heart and vascular diseases, such as coronary artery disease, congestive heart failure, myocardial infarction, and more. As medical-surgical nurses, your role extends far beyond simple disease management. It involves active participation in the diagnosis, treatment plan formulation, post-operative care, patient education, rehabilitation, and supportive care.

Our exploration of cardiovascular nursing begins with the essential basics: anatomy and physiology of the heart and vascular system. This foundational knowledge will guide us as we delve further into the domain. It will give us the keys to understanding the intricate balance of pressures, volumes, and electrical impulses that govern these systems.

Next, we explore common cardiovascular disorders and diseases, their pathophysiology, and their implications on patients' health. Here, we start understanding the complexities involved in managing these conditions and the importance of our role as healthcare providers. Each disease is unique, and so is every patient. Learning to balance the treatment protocols with individual patient needs is a skill we strive to master as CMSRNs.

The ability to interpret diagnostic tests, like ECGs and angiograms, is another crucial facet of cardiovascular nursing. These tools provide the roadmap to understanding the patient's condition, guiding our subsequent management strategies.

This chapter also dives into the therapeutic interventions common in cardiovascular care. We'll explore surgical procedures, medications, lifestyle modifications, and non-pharmacological treatments that form the backbone of cardiovascular nursing care. Understanding the rationale behind each intervention equips us with the knowledge to be passive caregivers and active contributors to the patient's healthcare team.

Lastly, patient education and health promotion form the cornerstones of cardiovascular nursing. Through strategies such as smoking cessation, promoting physical activity, healthy eating, and medication adherence, we can impact our patients' lives.

Cardiovascular nursing is a vibrant, ever-evolving field, continually pushing us to learn, adapt, and grow as professionals. Through this chapter, we'll navigate the complexities and challenges of this field together, ultimately working towards our goal of becoming adept, well-rounded CMSRNs.

Heart and Vascular Diseases

We encounter a range of illnesses that might upset the body's complex equilibrium as we make our way through the maze of cardiovascular ailments. These conditions have a variety of manifestations, from coronary artery disease to heart failure, and each has a particular etiology and implications.

Coronary artery disease (CAD)

When the coronary arteries, which carry blood to the heart muscle, become blocked by plaque formation, a condition known as atherosclerosis, coronary artery disease, a significant cause of morbidity and mortality globally, results. Angina (chest pain) or a heart attack (myocardial infarction) are frequently brought on by the hardening and narrowing of the arteries caused by plaque.

Myocardial Infarction (MI)

A myocardial infarction, also called a heart attack, is a dangerous disorder in which a blood clot frequently unexpectedly blocks the blood flow to a portion of the heart. The heart's ability to pump blood can be harmed by a lack of blood supply to the heart muscle. Severe chest pain, breathlessness, perspiration, and nausea are possible symptoms. To prevent cardiac damage and preserve lives, prompt medical attention is essential.

Congestive Heart Failure (CHF)

The heart doesn't pump blood as well as it should be due to chronic heart failure (CHF). High blood pressure, a MI, or CAD disorders can cause the heart to work too hard. Breathlessness, exhaustion, swelling legs, and an accelerated heartbeat can all be symptoms. Although dangerous, CHF patients' quality of life can be considerably improved with early detection and appropriate therapy.

Arrhythmias

Arrhythmias are irregular heartbeats that can make the heart's pumping less efficient. Heart disease, stress, certain drugs, or heredity can cause arrhythmias, ranging in severity from life-threatening to harmless. Typical kinds include bradycardia, tachycardia, and atrial fibrillation. Medications, dietary changes, or implantable devices may all be used in treatment, depending on the condition's severity and kind.

Hypertension

Hypertension, often known as high blood pressure, is a chronic illness in which the blood's force against the artery walls is consistently too high. Serious side effects such as heart attack, stroke, and kidney failure might result if not treated. Regular blood pressure monitoring is crucial because hypertension frequently has no symptoms.

Peripheral Artery Disease (PAD)

Blood flow to the limbs is decreased in PAD, a cardiovascular ailment caused by constricted blood arteries. The risk of CAD, MI, and stroke can all be impacted by PAD, which is primarily brought on by atherosclerosis. Walking pain, numbness, and coldness in the lower legs are frequent symptoms.

Understanding these diseases is paramount for any aspiring CMSRN. It equips us with the knowledge to anticipate complications, address patient concerns, and advocate for comprehensive care plans. Remember, our goal as CMSRNs isn't merely to treat diseases; it's to treat people. And the more we understand these conditions, the better we can serve those afflicted.

Interventions and Treatments

Comprehending the subtleties of various procedures and treatments is as essential in cardiovascular nursing as learning the disorders themselves. The range of remedies for cardiovascular illnesses is wide and varied, including pharmaceutical medicines, lifestyle modifications, and surgical interventions.

Pharmacologic Therapies

The cornerstone of managing cardiovascular disease is pharmacologic treatment. Depending on the illness, different medication classes are utilized, each with specific processes.

- **Antiplatelets and anticoagulants:** These drugs prevent clot formation, essential in conditions like myocardial infarction or for patients with stents. Aspirin, clopidogrel, and warfarin are a few examples.
- **Beta-blockers:** Used to treat hypertension, heart failure, and post-MI management, these drugs lessen the workload on the heart by lowering heart rate and blood pressure.
- ARBs and ACE inhibitors relax and widen blood arteries, lowering blood pressure and easing the symptoms of heart failure.
- **Statins:** These medications that decrease cholesterol are essential for treating atherosclerosis and avoiding cardiovascular problems.

Surgical Interventions

Medication and lifestyle modifications may not be sufficient in some circumstances, necessitating surgical surgery.

- **Coronary Artery Bypass Grafting (CABG):** In CABG, surgeons create a new route for blood to reach the heart muscle, bypassing the blocked coronary artery. A small balloon is inflated inside the narrowed artery to open it up and allow blood to flow again. A stent is then inserted to maintain the passageway open.
- **Pacemakers and implantable cardioverter-defibrillators (ICDs):** In patients with severe arrhythmias, devices like pacemakers and ICDs can help control cardiac rhythm.

Lifestyle Modifications

Pharmaceutical and surgical procedures are frequently combined with lifestyle modifications to address cardiovascular disorders.

- **Dietary changes** can help manage weight, blood pressure, cholesterol, and blood sugar by focusing on heart-healthy foods like fruits, vegetables, lean proteins, and whole grains while reducing added sugars, salt, and saturated fats.
- **Physical activity:** Regular physical activity helps improve cholesterol levels, lower blood pressure, and enhance cardiovascular health. The workout program must be customized to the person's tastes and abilities.
- **Quitting smoking:** A significant risk factor for cardiovascular illnesses is smoking. Helping individuals quit smoking can significantly lower their chance of developing heart disease.
- **Stress reduction:** Long-term stress is linked to an increased risk of cardiovascular disease. Stress management methods include mindfulness, yoga, and other forms of relaxation.

Rehabilitation

A complete program for those suffering from a heart attack, heart failure, angioplasty, or heart surgery is called cardiac rehabilitation. It includes specialized fitness instruction, information on leading a heart-healthy lifestyle, and counseling to lessen stress and support getting back to an active lifestyle.

Heart Valve Surgery

Certain heart conditions like stenosis or regurgitation cause the heart valves to malfunction. To fix or replace these faulty valves, patients undergo heart valve surgery, significantly reducing their symptoms and improving their quality of life.

Heart Transplant

Patients with advanced heart failure may only receive this medication as a last option. A healthy heart from a deceased donor replaces the patient's failing heart in a heart transplant. Complex post-transplant care is required, including ongoing medication to avoid organ rejection and continuous monitoring.

Ventricular Assist Devices (VADs)

Mechanical pumps, known as VADs, assist a failing heart in pumping blood throughout the body. For patients who are unable to have a transplant, they can act as a stopgap measure or, in some circumstances, a permanent fix.

Medication Adherence

Medication adherence is one of the most important parts of controlling cardiovascular disease. As healthcare professionals, we must emphasize the need to routinely and properly take prescribed medications. This entails describing possible adverse effects and resolving any obstacles to adherence, like expense or challenging prescription regimes.

Patient and Family Education

Cardiovascular nursing places a high priority on educating patients and their families about their condition and available treatments. This can involve educating people on how to spot symptoms of a worsening disease, how to manage them, the value of keeping follow-up appointments, and how to improve their lifestyle.

End-of-Life Care

The emphasis may change from aggressive treatment to palliative care in advanced cardiac disease. This entails treating symptoms, enhancing quality of life, and assisting patients and their families as they cope emotionally with terminal illnesses. Approaching these situations sensitively and empathetically and providing resources for emotional and psychosocial assistance is crucial.

Continuing Research and Evidence-Based Practice

Cardiovascular nursing is a dynamic and ever-changing area. Keeping up with the most recent findings, novel therapies, and best practice recommendations is imperative. Because of our dedication to lifelong learning, we can offer our patients the most cutting-edge, efficient care.

Medical, surgical, and supportive techniques are all included in the full range of cardiovascular interventions and treatments. As nurses, we put these therapies into practice, keep track of patient reactions, and modify care plans as necessary. We are improving our capacity to deliver first-rate patient care, standing up for our patients, and contributing to better cardiovascular health outcomes by expanding our understanding of these therapies.

PULMONARY NURSING

Venturing forward in our exploration of medical-surgical nursing, we now arrive at another binding domain: Pulmonary Nursing. It's a realm that demands a comprehensive understanding of the respiratory system, its diseases, and innovative nursing strategies to combat them.

Pulmonary nursing revolves around caring for patients afflicted with respiratory disorders ranging from chronic obstructive pulmonary disease (COPD) to pneumonia, asthma, lung cancer, and beyond. As CMSRNs, our role isn't confined to disease management; we engage in patient assessment, education, intervention planning, and ongoing reassessment.

Our exploration begins with the **rudimentary**: the anatomy and physiology of the respiratory system. An in-depth understanding of the system's workings forms the foundation for recognizing the implications of disease and treatment effects. You'll learn about oxygen and carbon dioxide flow, the intricate mechanics of ventilation, and the essential function of gas exchange.

Next, we delve into the broad spectrum of pulmonary diseases. We'll explore their pathophysiology, symptoms, and complications. Understanding these disorders is pivotal as it equips us with the knowledge to anticipate and manage complications, answer patient queries, and advocate for comprehensive care.

An essential part of pulmonary nursing is learning to interpret diagnostic tests. Pulmonary function tests, chest X-rays, CT scans, and bronchoscopies provide invaluable insight into the patient's condition. We'll guide you through interpreting these tests, ensuring you're equipped to utilize these tools in your practice effectively.

Following this, we'll explore the wide-ranging interventions and treatments in pulmonary care. From bronchodilators and corticosteroids to oxygen therapy, chest physiotherapy, and surgical interventions, you'll learn about these treatments' rationale, potential side effects, and nursing considerations.

Lastly, but significantly, we'll emphasize patient education and health promotion. This includes teaching about smoking cessation, the importance of immunizations, breathing exercises, and inhalers and nebulizers. Patient education is a cornerstone of nursing, fostering independence and enhancing self-management in our patients.

Pulmonary nursing is an intricate, ever-evolving field that demands a commitment to continuous learning and adaptation. In this chapter, we'll navigate the complexities together, developing a solid understanding of pulmonary conditions and treatments. Our objective is to evolve into skilled CMSRNs, capable of providing high-quality care to our patients with respiratory disorders. With each step, we come closer to becoming the exceptional nurses we aspire to be.

Respiratory Disorders

Let's explore the complex web of respiratory illnesses that CMSRNs can face in practice. These conditions range greatly, including lung cancer, chronic obstructive pulmonary disease (COPD), asthma, pneumonia, and tuberculosis.

Chronic Obstructive Pulmonary Disease (COPD)

COPD is a long-term inflammatory lung condition that impairs lung airflow. Emphysema and chronic bronchitis are the two disorders that make up the majority of them. The main risk factor is smoking; common symptoms include shortness of breath, increased sputum production, and a persistent cough. Although COPD progresses, it can be effectively treated with medicine, oxygen therapy, and lifestyle changes.

Asthma

Chronic asthma is characterized by inflamed airways that can constrict in response to different triggers, making breathing difficult. Wheezing, shortness of breath, chest tightness, and coughing are symptoms. Even though there is no known cure, asthma can be effectively managed by avoiding triggers and using drugs like bronchodilators and inhaled corticosteroids.

Pneumonia

A pneumonia illness causes the air sacs in one or both lungs to become inflamed. Its symptoms include a productive cough, a fever, chills, and breathing difficulties. Bacteria, viruses, or fungi may bring it on. Depending on the etiological agent, the usual course of treatment includes antibiotics, antivirals, or antifungals, in addition to supportive care, including rest and fluids.

Tuberculosis (TB)

Mycobacterium tuberculosis, a severe and frequently fatal infectious illness, is the cause of TB. The lungs are the main organs affected. However, they can spread to other body areas. A chronic cough, night sweats, exhaustion, and weight loss are typical symptoms. A comprehensive treatment plan combining numerous antibiotics is necessary for TB.

Lung Cancer

One of the most common cancers to cause death is lung cancer, which typically affects smokers. A persistent cough, chest pain, hoarseness, weight loss, and shortness of breath can all be symptoms. Surgery, radiation therapy, chemotherapy, targeted therapy, and immunotherapy are all available as treatment options.

Pulmonary Embolism (PE)

PE is a sudden obstruction of a pulmonary artery, typically brought on by a blood clot originating in a lower leg. It might be fatal. Therefore, you should get medical help right now. Sudden breathlessness, chest pain, and cough are symptoms. Anticoagulants or thrombolytics are frequently used as a form of treatment to dissolve the clot.

Pulmonary Hypertension

A form of high blood pressure known as pulmonary hypertension affects the arteries in the lungs and the right side of the heart. Since the symptoms are frequently the same as those of other heart and lung problems, a thorough evaluation is necessary to make the diagnosis. Medication, oxygen therapy, and in extreme situations, surgery or transplantation may all be used as forms of treatment.

Cystic Fibrosis (CF)

Cystic fibrosis is a fatal hereditary condition that predominantly affects the digestive and respiratory systems. It is characterized by the accumulation of thick, sticky mucus, which can seriously harm these organs. Some symptoms include chronic coughing, recurrent lung infections, wheezing, shortness of breath, and poor growth or weight gain. Although there is no cure, treatment plans try to control symptoms and stop the condition from worsening.

Idiopathic Pulmonary Fibrosis (IPF)

The fibrotic (scarring) alterations in the lung tissue that induce stiffness and cause severe dyspnea and coughing are the hallmarks of IPF, a chronic, progressive lung disease. Often, there is no recognized reason (thus the term "idiopathic"). Even though there is presently no treatment for IPF, several drugs can sometimes halt the disease's progression.

Sarcoidosis

Granulomas, aberrant clusters of inflammatory cells, can develop in various organs, including the lungs, due to sarcoidosis. Cough, breathlessness, and chest pain are all possible pulmonary symptoms. Even though there is no cure, most sarcoidosis patients receive little to no treatment and go about their daily lives.

Sleep Apnea

Frequent pauses characterize a sleep ailment called sleep apnea, and start breathing while you're asleep. Loud snoring and feeling exhausted even after a night's sleep are symptoms. Heart disease and stroke are two severe outcomes of untreated sleep apnea.

Pleural Effusion

An abnormal fluid buildup in the pleural space, the region between the layers of tissue lining the lungs and chest cavity, is known as a pleural effusion. Various illnesses, including pneumonia, lung cancer, or heart failure, may bring it on. Shortness of breath, a dry cough, and chest pain are symptoms. The fluid may be drained, or the source of the effusion may be addressed as part of the treatment, which focuses on the underlying cause.

Pneumothorax

When air seeps into the area between the chest wall and the lung, wholly or partially, the result is a pneumothorax or collapsed lung. This may happen voluntarily or as a result of an injury. Shortness of breath and abrupt chest discomfort are symptoms. The course of treatment might range from surveillance to urgent measures like inserting a chest tube.

To sum up, CMSRNS must thoroughly grasp these respiratory illnesses to deliver high-quality care. We can successfully monitor patients, foresee difficulties, and educate patients and their families by simply understanding their pathophysiology, symptoms, diagnostics, and treatment options. With every disorder we master, our knowledge, self-assurance, and the care we offer improve.

Interventions and Treatments

Now that we have a thorough grasp of these conditions let's focus on the strategies and therapies CMSRNs use to manage respiratory problems.

Pharmacologic Treatments

A lot of the time, pharmaceutical interventions serve as our first line of defense. Breathing becomes more accessible because bronchodilators like albuterol and tiotropium widen the airways. Corticosteroids and other anti-inflammatories lessen edema in the airways. Infections are treated with antibiotics and antivirals, whereas pulmonary embolism is treated with anticoagulants and thrombolytics.

Oxygen Therapy

Another essential treatment is oxygen therapy, especially for conditions like COPD and pneumonia that lead to hypoxemia. Masks, nasal cannulas, and non-invasive ventilation are all options for delivering oxygen. Monitoring oxygen levels and adjusting therapy as needed are crucial.

Breathing Techniques

Patients with COPD and asthma who use breathing techniques like pursed-lip and diaphragmatic breathing can better control their symptoms. These approaches can lessen dyspnea and enhance gas exchange by decreasing the rate of breathing and ensuring complete exhalation.

Pulmonary Rehabilitation

Programs for pulmonary rehabilitation can significantly enhance the quality of life for those with chronic lung diseases. They frequently include nutrition guidance, fitness instruction, education, and counseling.

Surgical Interventions

Surgery may be needed in situations that are severe or refractory. Lung volume reduction, bullectomy, and lung transplantation are all life-saving procedures. However, they come with significant hazards and necessitate cautious patient selection.

Patient Education

As nurses, we must educate patients. This can be imparting knowledge on the value of immunizations, quitting smoking, using inhalers effectively, or knowing when to seek medical treatment.

Palliative Care

Palliative care must also be considered. Some respiratory conditions, such as advanced COPD, IPF, or lung cancer, can significantly impact the quality of life. A multidisciplinary team is involved in palliative care to address the patient's needs as a whole person. Its goals include symptom relief, distress management, and quality of life enhancement.

Nebulizer Treatments

Nebulizers are devices used to administer medications in the form of a mist inhaled into the lungs. They're frequently used when a patient needs a higher dosage of drugs, when they can't use an inhaler correctly, or when a speedy reaction is necessary, like during an acute asthma attack. Nebulizers are frequently used to provide bronchodilators and corticosteroids.

Chest Physiotherapy

Using methods including percussion, vibration, and postural drainage, chest physiotherapy (CPT) helps patients cough up mucus that has become loose in their lungs. Patients with cystic fibrosis, COPD, or pneumonia may benefit from CPT.

Positive Pressure Ventilation

Positive pressure ventilation could be necessary in cases of severe respiratory failure. This could entail invasive procedures like mechanical ventilation or non-invasive techniques like continuous positive airway pressure (CPAP) and bilevel positive airway pressure (BiPAP). These therapies necessitate close observation for potential side effects, such as pneumothorax or ventilator-associated pneumonia.

Tracheostomy Care

A tracheostomy, a surgically made hole through the front of the neck into the trachea, may be required for individuals with long-term ventilatory demands. CMSRNs must be knowledgeable about providing tracheostomy care, which entails suctioning, cleaning, replacing the tracheostomy tube, and checking for issues like infection or blockage.

Smoking Cessation Programs

Smoking cessation is essential to respiratory healthcare since it reduces the risk of numerous respiratory disorders, including lung cancer and COPD. Counseling, drugs like varenicline or bupropion, and nicotine replacement therapy may all be used in this situation.

Vaccinations

Infections in the respiratory system, such as influenza and pneumococcal pneumonia, which can be severe or even fatal in people with pre-existing lung disorders, must be prevented by vaccinations. As CMSRNs, we are responsible for guaranteeing that our patients are immunized to date.

End-of-Life Care

End-of-life care becomes a critical management component for terminal illnesses such as advanced lung cancer or severe IPF. Assuring patient comfort, attending to psychosocial needs, and enabling conversations regarding advance care planning are all part of this.

As CMSRNs, it is our responsibility to provide compassionate care that is individualized to each patient's requirements while utilizing evidence-based interventions and treatments. It's a demanding job but immensely rewarding since we can significantly impact the lives of those we care for.

GASTROINTESTINAL NURSING

Welcome to the dynamic world of gastrointestinal nursing, a specialty that puts us at the forefront of patient care for various digestive system disorders. As Certified Medical-Surgical Registered Nurses (CMSRNs), we need to be equipped with a robust understanding of the gastrointestinal (GI) system and the diseases that may afflict it.

The GI system is a complex network stretching from the mouth to the anus, including the esophagus, stomach, small intestine, large intestine, rectum, liver, gallbladder, and pancreas. Each section has a distinct role in the digestion and absorption of nutrients, making the GI system vital for overall health.

In GI nursing, our patients can suffer from a wide variety of conditions. These can range from joint disorders like gastroesophageal reflux disease (GERD) and peptic ulcer disease to inflammatory conditions like Crohn's disease and ulcerative colitis to life-threatening diseases like liver cirrhosis and colorectal cancer. Understanding these conditions, their symptoms, complications, and treatment options is essential in providing high-quality care.

Patient care in GI nursing extends beyond addressing physical symptoms. We often assist with diagnostic procedures like endoscopies and colonoscopies, providing pre-procedure education, post-procedure monitoring, and comfort care. We also play a critical role in surgical procedures, from preoperative preparation to post-operative recovery and rehabilitation.

A key component of our role is educating patients about lifestyle modifications to manage or prevent GI diseases. This could involve diet changes, stress management techniques, medication compliance, or smoking and alcohol cessation. We often work in multidisciplinary teams with dieticians, therapists, and pharmacists, among others, to ensure comprehensive patient care.

Finally, the psychosocial aspects of GI diseases should not be overlooked. Conditions like irritable bowel syndrome (IBS) and inflammatory bowel disease (IBD) can significantly impact patients' quality of life, leading to anxiety or depression. Here, our role extends to providing emotional support, assisting in managing mental health issues, and referring to mental health professionals when necessary.

In summary, gastrointestinal nursing is an exciting and diverse field, requiring a broad skillset and the ability to provide holistic, patient-centered care. As CMSRNs, we aim to treat the disease and respect the entire person, advocating for their health and well-being at every step. As we delve deeper into this chapter, we will expand our understanding of the gastrointestinal system, its diseases, and our pivotal role in managing these conditions. Our journey into gastrointestinal nursing begins here. Let's move forward equipped with the curiosity, empathy, and desire to make a meaningful difference in our patients' lives.

Digestive Disorders

We CMSRNs deal with a variety of digestive issues. Let's get started with the common diseases that gastrointestinal nurses may encounter.

Gastroesophageal Reflux Disease (GERD)

Acid from the stomach commonly runs back into the esophagus, the tube that connects the mouth and stomach, leading to the chronic condition known as GERD. The lining of the esophagus may become inflamed from this acid reflux. Heartburn, acid regurgitation, and swallowing issues are typical symptoms.

Peptic Ulcer Disease (PUD)

PUD is characterized by sores or ulcers that form on the lining of the esophagus, upper small intestine, or stomach. Infection with the Helicobacter pylori bacterium or chronic use of nonsteroidal anti-inflammatory medicines (NSAIDs) are the leading causes of PUD. Symptoms can include nausea, bloating, and scorching stomach discomfort.

Gastritis

Inflammation of the stomach lining is called gastritis. Several conditions can bring it on, such as an H. pylori infection, persistent bile reflux, and routine NSAID use. Acute or chronic gastritis may develop rapidly (acute gastritis), and in some circumstances, it can cause ulcers and raise the risk of stomach cancer.

Inflammatory Bowel Disease (IBD)

IBD refers to a set of gastrointestinal conditions, the most prevalent of which are Crohn's disease and ulcerative colitis, that result in persistent digestive tract inflammation. IBD can be extremely painful and occasionally cause life-threatening complications. Diarrhea, stomach pain, exhaustion, and weight loss are possible symptoms.

Irritable Bowel Syndrome (IBS)

Irritable bowel syndrome (IBS) is a common condition that affects the large intestine and results in cramping, stomach pain, bloating, gas, diarrhea, and constipation as symptoms. Contrary to inflammatory bowel illness, which can be painful, IBS doesn't alter intestinal tissue or raise the risk of colon cancer.

Gallstones

Gallstones are consolidated deposits in the gallbladder that can be painful and cause digestive issues. They develop when elements in the bile, the digestive fluid, solidify. Gallstones can result in problems such as bile duct blockage, which can result in inflammation and infection.

Hepatitis

The most frequent cause of liver inflammation, known as hepatitis, is a viral infection. Hepatitis viruses come in five basic categories: A, B, C, D, and E. Cirrhosis or liver cancer can result from chronic hepatitis, especially hepatitis B and C.

Cirrhosis

Cirrhosis is a late stage of liver scarring (fibrosis) brought on by various liver disorders and conditions, including prolonged alcoholism and hepatitis. A potentially fatal disease called liver failure can result from cirrhosis.

Pancreatitis

Pancreatitis is an inflammation of the pancreas that can manifest as either an acute condition that manifests suddenly and lasts for days or a chronic disease that develops gradually over many years.

Colorectal Cancer

Cancer that develops in the colon or rectum is called colorectal cancer. Small, benign cell clusters called polyps are usually where it starts; over time, they can become malignancies.

These are only a handful of the digestive issues we, as CMSRNs, could face in practice. Each illness has different difficulties and necessitates another method of management and treatment. To provide ourselves with the knowledge we need to deliver top-notch, patient-centered care, we will further explore these conditions' etiology, diagnosis, and management as we progress through this chapter.

Diverticular Disease

Diverticula, tiny bulging pouches that grow in the digestive system's lining, indicate diverticular illness. Although they can develop anywhere in your digestive system, they frequently do so in the lower portion of the large intestine. Diverticulitis can result from these inflamed or infected pouches and cause excruciating stomach pain, fever, and bowel abnormalities.

Celiac Disease

In the case of celiac disease, eating gluten causes damage to the small intestine. In the entire world, one in every hundred persons is thought to be affected. The body has difficulty absorbing nutrients, particularly fat, calcium, iron, and folate, due to damage to the intestine.

Gastroenteritis

Gastroenteritis, also referred to as stomach flu, is an infection with a virus, bacteria, or parasite that causes the lining of the intestines to inflame. Dehydration may arise from the extreme diarrhea and vomiting that it causes.

Anal Fissures

A small rip in the mucosa, a delicate, moist tissue that lines the anus, is known as an anal fissure. This could happen when you pass huge or complicated feces during a bowel movement. Anal fissures frequently result in discomfort and bleeding during bowel movements.

Hemorrhoids

Veins in the lowest portion of your rectum and anus that are inflamed are called hemorrhoids. Sometimes, especially during bowel motions, the walls of these blood vessels stretch so thinly that the veins enlarge and become irritating.

To properly monitor and treat these illnesses, we must be competent and organized in our nursing practices. Our healthcare team members aim to deliver a high-quality treatment plan that attends to the patient's physical and emotional requirements. The interventions might be anything from giving emotional support and instruction to undergoing medical procedures, dietary changes, and lifestyle adjustments.

The specifics of these interventions and treatments, essential for favorable patient outcomes, are covered in the following section. In our responsibilities as CMSRNs, the value of thorough knowledge and compassionate patient care cannot be stressed.

Our fundamental goal is still to enhance our patient's quality of life and advance their health literacy so that they are better equipped to manage their health. Let's keep in mind our crucial role in the health of our patients as we learn more about these conditions.

Interventions and Treatments

Our primary responsibility as CMSRNs is to offer patients with gastrointestinal problems evidence-based care. Examine the various approaches and procedures necessary for patient recovery and disease care.

Pharmacological Interventions

There are many different drugs for digestive issues available in the pharmaceutical industry. Acid-related diseases like GERD and peptic ulcer can be controlled with antacids, proton pump inhibitors (PPIs), and H2 blockers. Doctors recommend anti-inflammatory medications, immune system suppressants, and antibiotics for conditions like IBD and gastritis. Antiviral treatments treat hepatitis, whereas pills to dissolve gallstones may be administered. Supplements for fiber, laxatives, anti-diarrheal, anticholinergic, antispasmodic, and antidepressant drugs are among the pharmaceuticals used to treat irritable bowel syndrome. Nurses need to be aware of the adverse effects and contraindications of each drug.

Surgical Interventions

Surgery could be required for some illnesses. Laparoscopic surgeries, the least intrusive procedure, and significant operations are possible. For instance, a cholecystectomy (gallbladder removal) may be necessary in severe gallstone situations. For early-stage malignancies, surgical treatments for colorectal cancer range from polypectomy and local excision to colectomy for more advanced problems. Surgery to remove damaged digestive tract tissue may be required in challenging IBD cases. Significant or persistent hemorrhoids may require a hemorrhoidectomy. In these situations, it is essential to understand preoperative and postoperative treatment.

Dietary Interventions

Many gastrointestinal problems can be effectively managed with diet. Smaller meals, avoiding food triggers, and not eating right before bedtime may be advised to patients with GERD; a low residue or low FODMAP diet may be suggested to people with IBD or IBS. An absolute lifelong gluten-free diet is required for people with celiac disease. As nurses, we can help patients' symptoms and quality of life by educating them about proper dietary modifications.

Lifestyle Modifications

Promoting healthy lifestyle modifications among patients can significantly impact how gastrointestinal problems are managed. Results can be enhanced by regular exercise, maintaining a healthy weight, quitting smoking, consuming less alcohol, and learning stress management skills.

Therapeutic Procedures

Some conditions might need therapeutic measures. For instance, paracentesis may be necessary for individuals with cirrhosis to reduce ascites-related abdominal pressure. Patients with severe pancreatitis may require necrosectomy or pancreatic duct drainage. It is crucial to comprehend the care needed for these treatments.

Palliative Care

Palliative Care (PC): For patients with terminal illnesses like advanced liver disease or colorectal cancer, PC aims to relieve symptoms and enhance the quality of life. This could include end-of-life care, nutritional support, psychological support, and pain management.

Patient Education

As nurses, one of our most important responsibilities is to impart knowledge. Patients must know their diseases, treatment plans, dietary restrictions, and lifestyle changes. Additionally, they must be mindful of the indications and symptoms that demand urgent medical attention. Our objective is to give them the tools to manage their diseases and take charge of their health effectively.

Our function as gastrointestinal nurses is varied. To provide comprehensive, patient-centered care, we must stay current on the most recent therapies and interventions and comprehend the consequences of various therapeutic alternatives.

Ultimately, it boils down to guiding our patients through their health journeys. One therapy or intervention at a time, the beauty of nursing is in the difference we make in the lives of our patients.

In the following chapters, we will go into more detail about other essential elements of medical-surgical nursing connected to the CMSRN exam, including endocrine, renal, and neurological nursing. Let's continue to remind ourselves of the significance of these therapies and interventions in our routine clinical work and how they affect our patients' overall well-being and quality of life.

Keep in mind that as CMSRNs, we also play an essential role in our patient's health journeys as educators, advocates, and caregivers. So let's arm ourselves with the knowledge and abilities we need to flourish in our professions and provide the best care possible for those in our care.

It could be challenging to become a CMSRN, but the work is worthwhile. Here's to a fruitful nursing career in medicine and surgery!

RENAL AND URINARY NURSING

Renal and urinary nursing, a specialized branch of medical-surgical nursing, centers around caring for patients with kidney and urinary system disorders. As a CMSRN candidate, you must thoroughly understand the functioning of these systems, various disease processes, their symptoms, and the subsequent nursing interventions and treatments.

The kidneys are workhorses in our bodies, performing a multitude of vital functions. They filter waste products, excess water, and other impurities from the blood. These waste products are stored in the bladder and eventually expelled through urination. Additionally, the kidneys regulate pH, salt, and potassium levels in our bodies, produce hormones affecting the function of other organs, and play a critical role in regulating blood pressure.

As renal and urinary nurses, we may encounter a range of conditions, from acute kidney injury (AKI), chronic kidney disease (CKD), urinary tract infections (UTIs), kidney stones, nephrotic syndrome, glomerulonephritis to more severe conditions like renal cancer.

Each of these disorders presents its unique challenges and requires specific care. For instance, in patients with CKD, our focus is often on managing the underlying causes like diabetes and hypertension, preventing the progression of kidney disease, and mitigating complications like anemia and bone disease. On the other hand, caring for a patient with a UTI often revolves around infection control and relief from painful symptoms.

One significant area under our responsibility is educating patients about their conditions, treatment options, potential lifestyle modifications, and preventative measures. This could involve teaching patients with recurrent kidney stones about the importance of hydration, a low-sodium, low-oxalate diet, and regular follow-ups to monitor their condition.

Furthermore, renal and urinary nurses play an instrumental role in caring for patients requiring renal replacement therapies, such as hemodialysis or peritoneal dialysis. Our position could involve everything from assessing vascular access, monitoring the dialysis process, and managing potential side effects to providing emotional support to patients and their families.

The beauty of nursing lies in its holistic approach. We're not merely addressing physical ailments but caring for our patient's emotional, mental, and social well-being. In renal and urinary nursing, we can make a real difference in our patient's quality of life.

In the upcoming sections, we'll delve deeper into the various renal and urinary disorders, their clinical manifestations, and the subsequent nursing interventions and treatments. Armed with this knowledge, we can provide exceptional patient-centered care, effectively manage our patient's health conditions, and contribute positively to their health journey. Let's continue our journey toward becoming competent CMSRNs!

Kidney and Urinary Tract Disorders

We start by learning about the many illnesses that might impact the renal and urogenital systems. Our nursing practice is built on an understanding of these disorders, enabling us to deliver efficient care specific to each patient's needs.

Acute Kidney Injury (AKI)

Acute kidney injury (AKI), formerly known as acute renal failure, is defined by a sudden decline in kidney function, which is frequently brought on by a severe injury, sickness, or medicine. It may cause the body's waste to build up harmfully. Clinical symptoms include reduced urine production and fluid retention that causes edema, weariness, and confusion. Early diagnosis and treatment of AKI can frequently stop developing chronic kidney disease (CKD).

Chronic Kidney Disease (CKD)

In CKD, kidney function gradually declines over time. It frequently results from diabetes, high blood pressure, or a family history of kidney disease. Anemia, weakness, weariness, and changes in urine output are typical symptoms. End-stage renal disease (ESRD), which calls for dialysis or kidney transplantation, may develop due to CKD.

Urinary Tract Infections (UTIs)

UTIs can affect any region of the urinary system, although the bladder and urethra are the most frequently affected. They are more common in women and are commonly brought on by bacteria. A typical symptom is a lower abdomen ache, frequent urination, and pain or burning while urinating. UTIs are often resolved with prompt antibiotic treatment. However, recurrent UTIs may require additional research.

Kidney Stones

When elements in the urine, such as calcium, oxalate, and phosphorus, concentrate to a high level, kidney stones might develop. The stones moving through the urinary tract may cause excruciating discomfort. Treatment options can include pain management, hydration intake, and surgery for more giant rocks.

Glomerulonephritis

This phrase describes conditions that harm the glomeruli, the kidneys' filtering organs. Glomerulonephritis can be acute or chronic, alone or in conjunction with another illness like lupus. Due to the presence of red blood cells or an abundance of protein, it might make urine frothy or turn pink or cola-colored.

Polycystic Kidney Disease (PKD)

A hereditary condition known as the development of many kidney cysts characterizes PKD. Over time, these cysts may impair renal function and result in kidney failure. High blood pressure, side or back pain, and abdominal fullness are typical symptoms.

Renal Artery Stenosis

This disorder causes the renal arteries, which carry blood to the kidneys, to constrict. It is most frequently brought on by atherosclerosis or fibromuscular dysplasia, and if left untreated, it can result in hypertension and renal damage.

Bladder Disorders
Bladder problems can range from bladder cancer to interstitial cystitis, a persistent ailment that causes pressure and pain in the bladder. Lower abdominal pain, frequent urination, and occasionally hematuria are common symptoms.

Nephrotic Syndrome
Due to this severe renal condition, the body excretes too much protein in the urine. Foamy urine, ankle, foot swelling, and weight increase from fluid retention are symptoms. It frequently results from harm to your kidneys' glomeruli, which are collections of microscopic blood veins.

Hydronephrosis
This illness is identified by the swelling of one or both kidneys due to an accumulation of urine. A blockage in the urinary tract, which prevents urine from flowing from the kidneys into the bladder, is a common cause of this condition. Fever, changes in urine, and side and back pain are possible symptoms.

Urinary Incontinence
In this, bladder control is lost, causing unintentional urine leaking. Mild leaking to unmanageable soaking are both possible. Urinary incontinence may be transient or persistent, depending on the underlying medical issue.

Renal Cell Carcinoma (R.C.C.)
The most typical kind of kidney cancer is RCC. It typically starts in the kidney's tubules, which are tiny tubes. It's frequently caught early and commonly affects older persons. Most RCC patients are asymptomatic in the early stages of the disease.

Vesicoureteral Reflux (VUR)
Due to this disease, urine might go backward from the bladder into the kidneys. The most common age groups for diagnosis are children and newborns. If left untreated, this can result in recurrent urinary tract infections and kidney harm.

Pyelonephritis
The bacteria that cause this kind of kidney infection typically arise from the bladder. If the germs get into the bloodstream, it can result in severe consequences such as high fever, back pain, and frequent urination.

Interstitial Cystitis (IC)
IC, also referred to as painful bladder syndrome, is a chronic illness that causes pelvic pain occasionally, as well as bladder pressure and pain. Mild discomfort to severe agony are all possible levels of pain. The condition belongs to a group of illnesses called painful bladder syndrome.

Prostatitis
The prostate gland, a walnut-sized gland that contributes to the fluid in semen and controls men's urination, is swollen and inflamed in this condition. It may result in frequent urination, groin pain, and sexual issues.

These are only a handful of conditions that might harm the urinary system and kidneys. We'll examine each condition's unique clinical manifestations, diagnostic techniques, and related nursing interventions and therapies as we go deeper into each. This knowledge will make our ability to successfully treat our patient's symptoms and enhance their quality of life possible. We are getting closer to being competent CMSRNs with each stage.

Interventions and Treatments

Understanding and using different intervention techniques and treatment modalities to address kidney and urinary tract problems is one of the most essential duties in renal and urinary nursing. Medical, surgical, and supportive treatments are necessary for these illnesses, which range from vesicoureteral reflux and urine incontinence to acute kidney damage and chronic kidney disease. The best patient outcomes and improved quality of life depend on understanding and using these treatments in a way that is appropriate to the illness and the patient's individual needs. The common interventions and treatments for a wide range of renal and urinary problems are covered in this part, giving medical-surgical nurses the information they need to provide patients with high-quality care.

Treatment Strategies for Acute Kidney Injury (AKI)

Treatment of the underlying cause and management of consequences are the main components of managing AKI to stop additional kidney damage. Medication, dialysis, and workplace hazards, including hypertension that can exacerbate AKI, are also possible forms of intervention. To avoid fluid overload, it is crucial to control fluid intake.

Management of Chronic Kidney Disease (CKD)

Addressing the root cause, this focuses on reducing the course of kidney disease. This can entail controlling blood sugar levels and blood pressure, making lifestyle adjustments, using drugs, and perhaps even getting a kidney transplant or sophisticated dialysis.

Approaches for Polycystic Kidney Disease (PKD)

Although PKD cannot be cured, therapy can lessen symptoms and avoid consequences. A kidney transplant, lifestyle modifications, pain treatment, hypertension control, cyst removal surgery, or any of these may be required.

Managing Glomerulonephritis

The main objective is to shield the kidneys from additional harm. Medication to lower blood pressure, reduce swelling, suppress immune system activity, or treat kidney failure are possible treatments.

Interventions for Kidney Stones

Options may include painkillers, drinking lots of water, medical therapy to help kidney stones pass, or procedures like extracorporeal shock wave lithotripsy, percutaneous nephrolithotomy, or ureteroscopy to remove or break up larger stones, depending on the type, size, and location of the rocks.

Dealing with Nephrotic Syndrome

Medications are typically used to address this condition's symptoms while lowering blood pressure, edema, high cholesterol, and infection risk.

Hydronephrosis Management

The goal of treatment is to remove urine from the kidneys. This can need a catheter, surgery to remove the obstruction, or medication to treat infection and pain.

Managing Urinary Incontinence

Treatment is based on the incontinence's kind, degree, and underlying cause. It may be as straightforward as behavioral approaches, bladder training, double voiding, scheduled bathroom visits, fluid and diet management, or more severe cases, it may call for drugs, medical equipment, or surgery.

Interventions for Renal Cell Carcinoma (RCC)

Nephrectomy surgeries, immunotherapy, targeted therapy, and radiation therapy are all included in this treatment.

Vesicoureteral Reflux (V.U.R.) Treatment

Antibiotics prevent UTIs; surgery may be necessary to repair the urinary tract's flaw.

Pyelonephritis Interventions

Antibiotics and, occasionally, hospitalization are frequently needed to treat this ailment.

Interstitial Cystitis (IC.) Management

Although there is no known treatment for IC, its symptoms can be controlled with drugs that help maintain the bladder's normal function, with physical therapy that eases pelvic pain, with nerve stimulation, and occasionally with surgery.

Prostatitis Treatment

Prostatitis can be treated with antibiotics, analgesics, alpha-blockers, and in some instances, prostate massage, depending on the underlying reason.

Learning these treatment choices is essential for anyone aiming to get the CMSRN credential. They are a crucial component of renal and urinary nursing. Remember that improving a patient's overall quality of life is as important as addressing their symptoms.

NEUROLOGICAL NURSING

Neurological nursing, a specialized healthcare area, involves caring for patients suffering from nervous system disorders. This challenging field demands a solid understanding of neurological conditions and exceptional nursing skills to manage patients' complex needs.

The nervous system, comprising the brain, spinal cord, and peripheral nerves, governs our bodies' functions, behaviors, and responses to external stimuli. It's a world in itself, and when disorders arise within this intricate network, the consequences can be life-altering. Patients experiencing neurological conditions present a unique set of clinical challenges, from cognitive and physical impairments to emotional and behavioral changes. This calls for dedicated, specialized nursing care.

Neurological nursing includes working with patients suffering from a wide array of disorders. Stroke, arguably the most commonly encountered condition in this field, can cause devastating physical and cognitive deficits. Timely intervention and comprehensive rehabilitative care are crucial to helping patients regain their lost abilities.

Similarly, neurodegenerative disorders like Alzheimer's and Parkinson's, while not reversible, require focused nursing care to slow progression, manage symptoms, and maintain quality of life. Understanding the nuanced presentations of these conditions and their impact on patient's lives is central to delivering effective care.

In contrast, conditions like epilepsy, a disorder marked by recurrent seizures, demand a distinct skill set. Here, nurses must manage acute seizure episodes, educate patients about triggers, and administer and monitor anti-epileptic therapies.

Traumatic brain injuries (TBIs) and spinal cord injuries, often resulting from accidents or falls, are other conditions that neurological nurses frequently encounter. These injuries can lead to a broad spectrum of impairments, from motor and sensory deficits to cognitive and emotional issues. The nursing care for these patients is multifaceted, addressing physical and mental rehabilitation and psychological support to help patients and their families adapt to a potentially changed life.

Neurological nurses also care for patients with brain tumors, multiple sclerosis, amyotrophic lateral sclerosis (ALS), Guillain-Barre syndrome, and many other complex neurological conditions. Each disorder necessitates a unique nursing approach guided by an understanding of the disease process and tailored to individual patient needs.

In addition to managing these conditions, neurological nurses play a significant role in preventive care. They educate patients and the public about risk factors for neurological diseases and promote lifestyle modifications to prevent these conditions.

Neurological nurses function as caregivers, educators, advocates, counselors, coordinators, and researchers in this multifaceted role. Their work is challenging but rewarding, making a profound difference in patients' lives. This chapter provides a deep dive into the field of neurological nursing, empowering you with the knowledge and skills you need to excel in this vital healthcare domain.

The subsequent sections will explore specific neurological disorders, their nursing management, and the interventions and treatments you should be proficient with as a CMSRN aspirant.

Neurological Disorders

Exploring the enormous world of neurological illnesses is like traversing a tricky maze. These diseases are numerous, and they can have a significant adverse effect on patients' life. This section explains the biology, symptoms, and consequences for patient care of some of the most prevalent neurological conditions.

Stroke

For nurses, a prevalent neurological disorder is a stroke, a medical emergency resulting from a blood clot (ischemic stroke) or a burst blood vessel (hemorrhagic stroke) that happens when blood flow to a particular brain area is disturbed. Because of the blood flow obstruction, brain cells are deprived of oxygen and perish. Patients may experience various symptoms, including paralysis, trouble speaking, memory loss, and behavioral abnormalities, depending on the location and degree of the stroke.

Epilepsy

The neurological disorder epilepsy, marked by recurring seizures, is also common. A quick, uncontrolled electrical surge in the brain causes seizures, manifesting symptoms ranging from momentary concentration lapses or muscular jerks to severe, protracted convulsions. The lifestyle, security, and mental well-being of an epilepsy patient can all be significantly impacted.

Neurodegenerative diseases

Progressive brain cell loss is a feature of neurodegenerative illnesses, including Alzheimer's and Parkinson's. The most prevalent dementia, Alzheimer's disease, causes memory loss, confusion, and mood swings. Parkinson's disease, on the other hand, primarily impacts motor function and manifests as tremors, rigidity, and balance issues. These chronic illnesses necessitate long-term nursing care that emphasizes symptom control, independence promotion, and quality of life preservation.

Multiple sclerosis (MS)

A chronic condition known as multiple sclerosis (MS) primarily affects the brain and spinal cord's ability to transmit messages. The symptoms of MS can range from weakness and trouble walking to numbness and impaired coordination. Nursing professionals have particular difficulties since MS symptom flare-ups are unpredictable.

Amyotrophic lateral sclerosis (ALS)

Lou Gehrig's disease, also known as amyotrophic lateral sclerosis (ALS), is a particular condition that affects nerve cells and pathways in the brain and spinal cord. Patients with ALS have a loss of muscle control and strength, making it difficult to speak, breathe, and swallow.

Guillain-Barre

Another severe condition, Guillain-Barre syndrome, is marked by the body's immune system wrongly attacking the peripheral nerves, causing weakness, numbness, and ultimately paralysis.

Traumatic brain injury (TBI)

Let's talk about traumatic brain injury (TBI), frequently brought on by jolts or vital strikes to the head. TBIs can cause many physical, mental, and behavioral symptoms, necessitating thorough, multidisciplinary care to promote healing and rehabilitation.

These conditions only comprise a small portion of the significant subject of neurology. The first step in giving patients with neurological disorders competent nursing care is understanding them, their distinctive manifestations, and how they affect patients' lives. The nursing care of these illnesses will be covered in more detail in later parts, along with examining the interventions and therapies employed to manage these disorders and direct patients toward the best results.

Interventions and Treatments

Given the variety of illnesses it deals with and the complexity of the nervous system, neurological nursing is a challenging area. But the available interventions and therapies have significantly improved due to developments in the medical sector. Here, we'll go over a few of them, emphasizing the diseases mentioned above.

Stroke Intervention and Treatment

A stroke is a medical emergency that has to be treated right away. The earlier treatment begins, the better the results because time is the brain. Stabilizing the patient's vital signs and using brain imaging to identify the type of stroke are the primary goals of the first therapy. The most frequent type of stroke, ischemic strokes, can be treated with thrombolytic medications that destroy the blood clot preventing blood flow to the brain. Surgery may be necessary for hemorrhagic strokes to relieve the strain brought on by the brain's bleeding.

Epilepsy Management

Anti-seizure drugs are the mainstay of treatment for epilepsy, with the selection being based on the type of seizures, the patient's age, potential adverse effects, and cost. Surgery, dietary therapy like the ketogenic diet, and nerve stimulation therapies may all be necessary in some circumstances.

Neurodegenerative Disease Management

Since there is no treatment for diseases like Alzheimer's and Parkinson's, these ailments rely on symptom control. Parkinson's and Alzheimer's disease include cognitive and motor symptoms that medication can control. Physical, occupational, and speech therapies can also aid the maintenance of function and quality of life.

Multiple Sclerosis (MS.) Treatment

The goals of MS therapy include managing symptoms, symptom management, and accelerating recovery following episodes. Options include corticosteroids for sudden attacks, pharmaceuticals that delay the advancement of the disease, and therapies that treat symptoms like exhaustion, trouble walking, and depression.

Amyotrophic Lateral Sclerosis (ALS.) Management

ALS treatment aims to reduce symptoms and enhance the quality of life. Medication can treat symptoms, including muscle stiffness, and delay the progression of the disease. Therapy tools and equipment for physical, occupational, and speech disorders can support independence and function.

Guillain-Barre Syndrome Treatment

Plasma exchange (plasmapheresis) and immunoglobulin therapy are the main treatments for Guillain-Barre Syndrome and work to lessen the intensity and duration of the immunological attack on the nerves. Physical medicine is also essential to regain strength and mobility throughout recovery.

Traumatic Brain Injury (TBI.) Management

Depending on the severity, TBI is treated in a variety of ways. It could entail rehabilitative therapy to restore lost skills, medicines to manage symptoms, and surgery to remove hematomas or fix fractures.

Migraine and Headache Management

Medications made to reduce symptoms and stop recurrences are frequently used to treat migraines and other headaches. A thorough treatment strategy must include non-pharmacological interventions like biofeedback, cognitive-behavioral therapy, and lifestyle changes, including getting enough sleep, drinking enough water, eating a healthy diet, exercising, and managing stress.

Spinal Cord Injury Treatment

Preventing additional harm and fostering the highest possible function and quality of life are the main objectives of managing spinal cord injuries. This may entail an emergency operation, rigorous physical therapy, and pain and spasticity medication. It's also essential to receive psychological treatment to deal with the emotional and mental health problems brought on by these permanently altering injuries.

Peripheral Neuropathy Management

The management of disease-producing peripheral neuropathy and symptom relief are the main goals of peripheral neuropathy treatment. Treatment varies depending on the underlying cause and can be as simple as managing diabetes or as complex as immunotherapy for autoimmune illnesses. Antidepressants, seizure medicines, and analgesics are frequently used to treat pain.

Neuromuscular Disorders Treatment

Comprehensive treatment plans are necessary for myasthenia gravis, muscular dystrophy, and spinal muscular atrophy. These plans include medications to increase muscle strength or slow muscle deterioration, physical therapy to maintain mobility and function, and supportive therapies to treat side effects like respiratory distress.

Sleep Disorders Management

To effectively treat sleep disorders, including insomnia, sleep apnea, and restless legs syndrome, lifestyle changes, CBT-I (cognitive behavioral treatment for insomnia), drugs, and equipment like CPAP machines are frequently used.

Neurological nursing covers various illnesses, each with its difficulties and available treatments. Nurses must stay current on the most recent research and treatment techniques to give their patients the best care possible as medical science advances. Understanding that each patient's path is distinct and calls for individualized care plans and compassionate care is vital.

MUSCULOSKELETAL NURSING

Musculoskeletal nursing opens up a vast knowledge that engages with the health and well-being of the human body's structural system. This branch of nursing explores the complexity of the muscles, bones, ligaments, tendons, and nerves that allow movement, shape, and stability to our bodies. For the aspiring CMSRN, mastery in this area is essential, as many patients require care due to musculoskeletal issues.

Musculoskeletal nursing encompasses many conditions, from fractures and sprains to chronic diseases such as osteoporosis and rheumatoid arthritis. These conditions can significantly impact a patient's quality of life, mobility, independence, and mental health.

Therefore, the role of the musculoskeletal nurse goes beyond physical care. These professionals are also involved in patient care's psychological, rehabilitative, and preventative aspects.

A musculoskeletal nurse's responsibilities are diverse and crucial. They are involved in assessing and managing pain, promoting mobility, administering and managing medication, and collaborating with the multidisciplinary team to provide holistic care. Additionally, they play a key role in patient education, equipping patients with the knowledge and tools to manage their conditions and prevent complications.

An integral part of musculoskeletal nursing is rehabilitation. Following an injury or surgery, patients often require a personalized rehabilitation plan to restore function, enhance mobility, alleviate pain, and improve quality of life. Nurses work closely with physiotherapists, occupational therapists, and other rehabilitation professionals to ensure patients regain the highest possible level of function.

In conclusion, musculoskeletal nursing is a challenging but rewarding field that demands a deep understanding of the human body's structural framework, a keen eye for assessment, and a compassionate approach to patient care. It offers a dynamic environment where nurses can continually learn, grow, and substantially impact patients' lives.

As you delve into the following sections, remember that the journey to becoming a successful musculoskeletal nurse starts with a solid foundation in understanding various musculoskeletal disorders and the treatments available for these conditions.

Musculoskeletal Disorders

Various illnesses that affect the body's musculoskeletal system are referred to as musculoskeletal disorders (MSDs). They range from sudden diseases like osteoarthritis and rheumatoid arthritis to persistent systemic conditions like fractures and sprains. Understanding these illnesses is essential for aspiring CMSRNs to provide patients with quality treatment.

Fractures
Fractures, the most frequent musculoskeletal condition, happen when excessive tension or force breaks a bone. Fractures can be simple (one perfectly aligned break) or complex (many frequently out of alignment). Repositioning the broken bone fragments, immobilizing the affected area with casts or splints, and in more challenging situations, surgical intervention is the conventional management technique. Exercises for rehabilitation and pain control are crucial to a patient's recovery.

Sprains and Strains

These are strains of the muscles or tendons and sprains of the ligaments. They frequently happen during athletic activities and are typically brought on by overstretching or ripping due to a rapid twist, pull, or impact. The RICE approach combines pain relief and physical therapy with rest, ice, compression, and elevation and is the cornerstone of treatment for many injuries.

Osteoarthritis (OA)

Osteoarthritis (O**A)** is a degenerative joint condition characterized by the slow loss of cartilage, which causes uncomfortable bone-on-bone contact. Knees, hips, and small hand joints are the most often impacted joints. Risk factors include aging, obesity, injuries, and heredity, even if the cause is unknown. Treatment aims to reduce pain, increase mobility, and improve quality of life. In severe situations, medication, physiotherapy, dietary changes, and joint replacement surgery accomplish this.

Rheumatoid Arthritis (RA)

In contrast to OA, RA is an autoimmune condition in which the body's immune system unintentionally assaults its tissues, most notably the synovium, the thin membrane that lines the joints. Joint deformity eventually results from it, along with joint swelling, discomfort, and inflammation. Although the precise origin of RA is unknown, a combination of genetic and environmental factors is involved. Medication to treat symptoms and slow the spread of the disease is part of management, along with physical therapy and occasionally surgery.

Osteoporosis

This bone condition makes frail bones more prone to breaking because of diminished bone density and strength. Since there may be no symptoms until a fracture occurs, it is frequently called a "silent disease." Age, family history, being underweight, smoking, and drinking too much alcohol are all risk factors. Treatment options include calcium and vitamin D supplements, drugs to reduce bone loss, weight-bearing workouts, and a diet suitable for the bones.

Musculoskeletal Back Pain

Problems with the muscles, ligaments, vertebrae, or spinal discs may cause this frequent disease. Poor posture, muscle strain, and severe disorders like ruptured discs or spinal stenosis are all potential causes. Depending on the source and extent of the pain, there are many different types of treatment, although physical therapy, medications, and dietary changes are frequently used. Surgery may be necessary in specific circumstances.

Gout

Gout is an inflammatory disorder that affects the joints and is brought on by the buildup of uric acid crystals. It frequently causes excruciating pain, redness, and swelling. Although the big toe is most commonly impacted, gout can affect any joint. The main treatment plan consists of dietary and lifestyle adjustments and drugs to reduce uric acid levels or control inflammation.

Fibromyalgia

The symptoms of this chronic condition include broad musculoskeletal discomfort, exhaustion, and painful spots in specific locations. Although the precise origin is unknown, it may be a combination of genetic, environmental, and psychological factors. The treatment uses various pharmaceuticals, physical activity, stress-reduction techniques, and good lifestyle choices.

Systemic Lupus Erythematosus (SLE)

SLE is a chronic autoimmune illness that affects the skin, joints, kidneys, heart, and lungs because the body's immune system mistakenly assaults healthy tissue. Common symptoms include stiffness and joint pain. Although SLE cannot be cured, its symptoms can be controlled with anti-inflammatory medicines, immunosuppressants, and dietary changes.

Tendinitis

Inflammation or irritation of a tendon is known as tendinitis, and it is frequently brought on by recurrent, minor trauma to the area in question or by sudden, more significant damage. The elbow, knee, shoulder, wrist, and heel are where it usually manifests itself. Physical therapy, painkilling drugs, resting the damaged area, and even surgery are all part of the course of treatment.

Carpal Tunnel Syndrome

The median nerve experiences pressure as it passes through the carpal tunnel in the wrist, resulting in this common ailment. The symptoms include numbness, tingling, and weakness in the hand and arm. Repetitive hand movements, pregnancy, and diseases, including rheumatoid arthritis and diabetes, are risk factors. Treatment options include wrist splinting, medication, and surgery for more severe cases.

In the extensive field of musculoskeletal nursing, comprehending these illnesses and their therapies is merely the tip of the iceberg. As you expand your understanding, keep in mind to concentrate on the clinical characteristics of these conditions, the methods of diagnosis, and the numerous therapeutic strategies that can reduce symptoms and enhance patients' quality of life. The following section will cover the therapies and treatments for these illnesses in more detail.

Interventions and Treatments

A thorough awareness of the numerous strategies and treatments that help patients manage their musculoskeletal problems is required for musculoskeletal nursing. Let's delve deeper into this topic and discuss how nurses can help patients improve.

Pain Management

Pain management becomes an essential component of the treatment strategy for many patients. It's common practice to take over-the-counter painkillers like acetaminophen (Tylenol), ibuprofen (Advil, Motrin), and naproxen sodium (Aleve). Doctors may recommend more potent painkillers in more severe cases. Patients must be closely observed by nurses to make sure their pain medications are working and to look out for any indications of side effects or dependence.

Physical Therapy and Rehabilitation

Numerous musculoskeletal problems are treated with physical therapy, which aims to strengthen the body, improve mobility, and lessen discomfort. Together with the nursing team, physical therapists develop patient-specific regimens. Nurses are essential in motivating patients to follow these regimens and keeping track of improvement.

Orthotic Devices

Braces, splints, and shoe inserts are orthotic devices that support weak joints and reduce pain. As a nurse, you'll frequently have to instruct patients on using these devices correctly and guarantee a suitable fit.

Surgical Interventions

Surgery could be necessary for musculoskeletal problems, such as severe fractures or joint abnormalities. As a nurse, you'll be essential in getting patients ready for surgery, keeping track of how they're doing afterward, managing their pain, and helping them recover and return to their old selves.

Lifestyle Modifications

Modifying one's way of life can significantly affect how musculoskeletal disorders are managed. Better results can be attained by promoting regular exercise, eating a balanced diet, and maintaining a healthy weight. Nurses frequently lead in implementing these adjustments and giving patients ongoing assistance and education.

Complementary Therapies

Complementary therapies, including acupuncture, massage, and mindfulness exercises, help many people. Although these therapies shouldn't be used in place of standard medical care, they can be a helpful addition.

Medication Management

Long-term pharmaceutical management is necessary for musculoskeletal disorders, including rheumatoid arthritis and osteoporosis. Drugs to lower inflammation, halt disease development, or increase bone density are frequently included. Nurses must thoroughly understand these medications, including any potential side effects, to monitor patients efficiently.

Patient Education

Educating patients about their diseases is a crucial part of musculoskeletal nursing. This includes describing the disease process, reviewing available treatments, showing patients exercises or employing orthotic devices, and responding to their inquiries. With the correct information, patients may actively participate in their healthcare decisions.

Psychosocial Support

For patients, managing chronic musculoskeletal disorders can be emotionally challenging. A nurse's role in holistic care includes the following:

- Offering emotional support.
- Assisting patients with their emotions.
- Linking them to mental health services.

Intravenous and Subcutaneous Therapies

Subcutaneous or intravenously injected medicines are sometimes utilized to treat musculoskeletal disorders. Biologics, frequently prescribed for diseases like rheumatoid arthritis, can be among them. As a nurse, you will assist with these therapies, watch out for adverse effects, and inform patients what to anticipate.

Occupational Therapy

Many people with musculoskeletal disorders require occupational therapy. It focuses on enhancing daily chores, such as getting dressed and cooking, as well as computer use and other work-related activities. You'll frequently work with occupational therapists to help patients integrate the techniques they've learned into their everyday routines.

Use of Heat and Cold

Musculoskeletal pain can be effectively managed with both heat and cold therapy. While cold therapy can reduce inflammation and numb discomfort, heat therapy can relax muscles and ease stiff joints. Instructing patients on how to use these treatments properly to prevent skin injury is essential.

Assistive Devices

Patients with musculoskeletal disorders can move much more easily using aids like wheelchairs, walkers, and canes. To prevent falls or injuries, you'll instruct patients on how to use these devices properly, ensure they're fitted correctly, and monitor how they're being used.

Joint Injections

Joint injections may be a solution for severe pain or inflammation. These can deliver potent anti-inflammatory medications right to the affected area. As a nurse, you'll prepare patients for the treatment, take care of them while they're recovering, and watch for any issues.

Advanced Surgical Interventions

Joint replacements or reconstructions may be required in extreme situations. As a nurse, you must assist with patient preparation, intraoperative and postoperative care, and rehabilitation. Additionally, you'll impart knowledge on how to care for wounds, avoid infections, and spot complications.

Comprehensive Pain Management

A thorough pain management strategy may be required for chronic musculoskeletal problems. To help patients manage their chronic pain, this can include pharmacological interventions, non-drug treatments like physical therapy or acupuncture, and psychological support.

Support Groups and Counseling

Patients with chronic musculoskeletal diseases need emotional and psychological assistance. You can point patients toward support groups so they can exchange stories and coping mechanisms. If necessary, you can also put them in touch with counseling services.

Preventive Care and Screening

Early diagnosis can have a substantial impact on the course of several musculoskeletal diseases. Regular screening and preventative treatment become essential, and you may contribute significantly to these proactive measures as a nurse.

PRACTICE TEST

Cardiovascular Nursing

1. What does the P wave signify on an electrocardiogram (ECG)?
    - **A)** Ventricular depolarization
    - **B)** Ventricular repolarization
    - **C)** Atrial depolarization
    - **D)** Atrial repolarization

2. Which of the following heart sounds signifies the closure of the mitral and tricuspid valves?
    - **A)** S1
    - **B)** S2
    - **C)** S3
    - **D)** S4

3. Which of the following is NOT a typical symptom of congestive heart failure (CHF)?
    - **A)** Edema
    - **B)** Fatigue
    - **C)** Bradycardia
    - **D)** Shortness of breath

4. What type of drug is nitroglycerin?
    - **A)** Anticoagulant
    - **B)** Vasodilator
    - **C)** Beta-blocker
    - **D)** Diuretic

5. Where is the apical pulse located?
    - **A)** At the 5th intercostal space at the left midclavicular line
    - **B)** At the 2nd intercostal space at the right sternal border
    - **C)** At the 2nd intercostal space at the left sternal border
    - **D)** At the 5th intercostal space at the right midclavicular line

6. Which lab value is NOT typically used to assess a patient's risk for heart disease?
    - **A)** Hemoglobin A1C
    - **B)** Cholesterol
    - **C)** Blood Urea Nitrogen (BUN)
    - **D)** Triglycerides

7. Which condition is a patient with a blood pressure reading of 150/95 mmHg likely to have?
    - **A)** Hypotension
    - **B)** Normal blood pressure
    - **C)** Prehypertension
    - **D)** Hypertension

8. What type of angina occurs unpredictably and might not be relieved by nitroglycerin or rest?
    - **A)** Stable angina
    - **B)** Unstable angina
    - **C)** Prinzmetal's angina
    - **D)** Microvascular angina

9. The nurse should teach a patient receiving digoxin therapy to report which of the following symptoms?
    A) Fatigue
    B) Visual disturbances such as yellow-green halos
    C) Diarrhea
    D) All of the above

10. Which heart failure classification describes a patient with symptoms at rest?
    A) Class I
    B) Class II
    C) Class III
    D) Class IV

11. What is the first line of treatment for a patient experiencing chest pain?
    A) Oxygen
    B) Aspirin
    C) Nitroglycerin
    D) Morphine

12. Which nursing intervention is appropriate for a patient who has just returned from cardiac catheterization?
    A) Encouraging the patient to ambulate
    B) Monitoring the patient's vital signs closely
    C) Applying warm compresses to the puncture site
    D) Administering a potassium supplement

13. What symptoms might you expect to find in assessing a patient with pericarditis?
    A) Distant, muffled heart sounds
    B) Decreased blood pressure
    C) Bradycardia
    D) Wheezing

14. A patient is receiving heparin therapy. Which lab value will the nurse monitor to evaluate the therapy's effectiveness?
    A) Prothrombin time (PT)
    B) Platelet count
    C) International normalized ratio (INR)
    D) Activated partial thromboplastin time (aPTT)

15. What are the three typical characteristics of pain related to myocardial ischemia?
    A) Dull, aching, and sharp
    B) Sudden onset, lasts 2-5 minutes and relieved with rest
    C) Substernal, radiating, and lasts longer than 30 minutes
    D) Sharp, burning, and relieved by changing position

16. Which of the following conditions is associated with left-sided heart failure?
    A) Peripheral edema
    B) Ascites
    C) Pulmonary edema
    D) Jugular vein distension

17. Which of the following is not a common risk factor for coronary artery disease (CAD)?
- **A)** Hypertension
- **B)** Smoking
- **C)** High HDL cholesterol levels
- **D)** Diabetes mellitus

18. Beta-blockers are used in managing heart failure primarily for their:
- **A)** Diuretic properties
- **B)** Ability to decrease heart rate and contractility
- **C)** Vasodilating properties
- **D)** Positive inotropic effects

Pulmonary Nursing

1. Which of the following is a common Chronic Obstructive Pulmonary Disease (COPD) symptom?
    A) Cough
    B) Wheezing
    C) Shortness of breath
    D) All of the above

2. Which type of breath sounds would you expect to hear in a patient with pneumonia?
    A) Crackles
    B) Wheezes
    C) Stridor
    D) Rhonchi

3. What is the primary cause of Respiratory Distress Syndrome (RDS) in premature infants?
    A) Pneumonia
    B) Asthma
    C) Lack of surfactant
    D) Allergic reaction

4. Which lung condition is characterized by the destruction of the walls of the alveoli, resulting in fewer, larger alveoli?
    A) Emphysema
    B) Asthma
    C) Bronchitis
    D) Pneumonia

5. What does the arterial blood gas (ABG) measurement PaCO2 reflect?
    A) The amount of oxygen in the blood
    B) The amount of carbon dioxide in the blood
    C) The blood's pH level
    D) The bicarbonate level in the blood

6. Which respiratory disorder is characterized by an overreaction of the tracheobronchial tree to various stimuli?
    A) Asthma
    B) Bronchitis
    C) Tuberculosis
    D) Emphysema

7. The Mantoux test is used to identify which disease.
    A) Asthma
    B) Pneumonia
    C) Tuberculosis
    D) Bronchitis

8. Which is NOT a common symptom of Tuberculosis (TB)?
    A) Chest pain
    B) Cough with blood-tinged sputum
    C) Wheezing
    D) Night sweats

9. The main goal of nursing care for a patient with pneumonia is:
    A) Minimize anxiety
    B) Maintain a clear airway
    C) Pain control
    D) Promote independence

10. Which patient behaviour increases the risk for lung cancer?
    A) High protein diet
    B) Smoking cigarettes
    C) Regular exercise
    D) Adequate sleep

11. Which of the following assessments would indicate a positive result for pleural effusion?
    A) Resonance heard on percussion
    B) Diminished breath sounds on the affected side
    C) Barrel-shaped chest
    D) Symmetrical chest expansion

12. A pulmonary function test measures:
    A) The capacity and function of the lungs
    B) The presence of lung disease
    C) The cause of shortness of breath
    D) All of the above

13. An acute asthma exacerbation would NOT typically result in which of the following?
    A) Wheezing on expiration
    B) Decreased respiratory rate
    C) Increased sputum production
    D) Use of accessory muscles for breathing

14. What is the primary nursing intervention for a patient suspected of having a pulmonary embolism?
    A) Encourage deep breathing and coughing
    B) Administer antipyretics
    C) Begin oxygen therapy
    D) Ambulate frequently

15. What assessment finding is characteristic of a patient with a tension pneumothorax?
    A) Decreased tracheal deviation
    B) Increased breath sounds on the affected side
    C) Decreased respiratory rate
    D) Hypotension

16. What is the primary therapeutic intervention for a Chronic Obstructive Pulmonary Disease (COPD) patient?
    A) Corticosteroid therapy
    B) Oxygen therapy
    C) Bronchodilator therapy
    D) Diuretic therapy

17. What is the primary side effect of theophylline?
    A) Hypertension
    B) Bradycardia
    C) Tachycardia
    D) Hypotension

18. What disease process is most commonly associated with the clubbing of the fingers?
    A) Asthma
    B) Pulmonary embolism
    C) Chronic hypoxia
    D) Pneumonia

Gastrointestinal Nursing

1. What is the primary function of the liver in digestion?
    A) Produce bile
    B) Secrete enzymes
    C) Absorb nutrients
    D) Store vitamins

2. Crohn's disease primarily affects which part of the gastrointestinal tract?
    A) Esophagus
    B) Stomach
    C) Small intestine
    D) Large intestine

3. Which symptom is NOT commonly associated with gastroesophageal reflux disease (GERD)?
    A) Dyspepsia
    B) Chest pain
    C) Diarrhea
    D) Regurgitation

4. A nurse should teach a patient with diverticulosis to avoid which of the following?
    A) High-fiber foods
    B) Adequate hydration
    C) Regular exercise
    D) Popcorn and seeds

5. Which of the following is a common cause of peptic ulcers?
    A) Helicobacter pylori infection
    B) High protein diet
    C) Lack of physical activity
    D) High-fiber diet

6. Which of the following is a risk factor for developing gallstones?
    A) Male gender
    B) Low-fat diet
    C) Obesity
    D) Regular exercise

7. What does the term 'steatorrhea' refer to?
    A) Blood in the stool
    B) Fatty stools
    C) Mucus in the stool
    D) Constipation

8. A patient with celiac disease should avoid foods containing which substance?
    A) Lactose
    B) Fructose
    C) Gluten
    D) Sucrose

9. The most common type of hernia in both men and women is:
    A) Umbilical hernia
    B) Incisional hernia
    C) Inguinal hernia
    D) Hiatal hernia

10. Which symptom is typically present in a patient with appendicitis?
    A) Right lower quadrant pain
    B) Left lower quadrant pain
    C) Right upper quadrant pain
    D) Left upper quadrant pain

11. What is the primary treatment for haemorrhoids?
    A) High-fiber diet
    B) Antacids
    C) Corticosteroids
    D) Surgery

12. Jaundice is a common symptom of which of the following conditions?
    A) Hepatitis
    B) Appendicitis
    C) Gastritis
    D) Ulcerative colitis

13. Which condition often presents with 'coffee-ground' vomitus?
    A) Peptic ulcer disease
    B) Gastroenteritis
    C) Irritable bowel syndrome
    D) Diverticulitis

14. What is the primary purpose of a nasogastric tube in a postoperative patient?
    A) Nutrition
    B) Hydration
    C) Decompression
    D) Medication administration

15. Which of the following is NOT a common cause of constipation?
    A) Inadequate fluid intake
    B) Inadequate fibre intake
    C) Overuse of laxatives
    D) Excessive exercise

16. What is a common complication of cirrhosis?
    A) Hypertension
    B) Ascites
    C) Hypoglycemia
    D) Hyperactivity

17. In a patient with pancreatitis, what would be an expected laboratory finding?
    A) Decreased amylase levels
    B) Increased amylase levels
    C) Decreased white blood cell count
    D) Increased red blood cell count

18. Esophageal varices are a common complication of which condition?
    A) Gastroenteritis
    B) Gastric ulcer
    C) Hepatitis C
    D) Cirrhosis

Renal and Urinary Nursing

1. Which of the following is a common sign of urinary tract infection (UTI)?
    A) Hematuria
    B) Hypertension
    C) Bradycardia
    D) Hyperglycemia

2. Which of the following is NOT a function of the kidney?
    A) Detoxification
    B) Regulation of blood pressure
    C) Production of insulin
    D) Regulation of electrolytes

3. Pyelonephritis is an infection of what part of the urinary system?
    A) Urethra
    B) Bladder
    C) Kidneys
    D) Ureters

4. Which of the following is a significant risk factor for developing kidney stones?
    A) Dehydration
    B) Low calcium intake
    C) Sedentary lifestyle
    D) High-fiber diet

5. Which of the following is a crucial symptom of glomerulonephritis?
    A) Polyuria
    B) Proteinuria
    C) Hypoglycemia
    D) Hypercalcemia

6. Renal failure can be categorized as acute or chronic. What is a distinguishing characteristic of chronic renal failure?
    A) Rapid onset
    B) Sudden loss of kidney function
    C) Long-standing disease
    D) Full recovery with treatment

7. What is the purpose of a urinary catheter?
    A) To deliver medication
    B) To remove urine from the bladder
    C) To filter the blood
    D) To measure blood pressure

8. What is polycystic kidney disease?
    A) A bacterial infection of the kidney
    B) A condition where multiple cysts develop in the kidneys
    C) An autoimmune disorder affecting the kidneys
    D) A malignant tumour in the kidneys

9. What is the primary function of dialysis in a patient with kidney failure?
    A) To stimulate kidney function
    B) To control blood pressure
    C) To filter toxins and waste from the blood
    D) To administer medication

10. A patient with end-stage renal disease (ESRD) might need which of the following treatments?
    A) Liver transplant
    B) Kidney transplant
    C) Lung transplant
    D) Heart transplant

11. What is a common symptom of bladder cancer?
    A) Hematuria
    B) Hyperglycemia
    C) Hypocalcemia
    D) Hypertension

12. What is the common cause of urinary incontinence in older adults?
    A) Overactive bladder
    B) Kidney stones
    C) Pyelonephritis
    D) Polycystic kidney disease

13. What diet is recommended for patients with chronic kidney disease to delay progression?
    A) Low-sodium, low-protein diet
    B) High-sodium, high-protein diet
    C) Low-carbohydrate, high-fat diet
    D) High-carbohydrate, low-fat diet

14. What medication is often prescribed to reduce proteinuria in patients with nephrotic syndrome?
    A) Beta-blockers
    B) Angiotensin-converting enzyme (ACE) inhibitors
    C) Diuretics
    D) Statins

15. Which of the following lab values would indicate decreased kidney function?
    A) Decreased creatinine clearance
    B) Increased glucose level
    C) Decreased blood urea nitrogen (BUN)
    D) Increased sodium level

16. A patient with hydronephrosis may have a history of which of the following conditions?
    A) Kidney stones
    B) Diabetes mellitus
    C) Hypertension
    D) Heart disease

17. What is a common early symptom of acute kidney injury (AKI)?
    A) Anuria
    B) Hypertension
    C) Hematuria
    D) Polyuria

18. Which type of urinary incontinence is due to overactivity of the detrusor muscles?
    A) Stress incontinence
    B) Urge incontinence
    C) Overflow incontinence
    D) Functional incontinence

Neurological Nursing

1. Which of the following is NOT a classic sign of Parkinson's disease?
    A) Tremor
    B) Rigidity
    C) Bradycardia
    D) Postural instability

2. Which of the following is the primary initial symptom in patients with multiple sclerosis?
    A) Fatigue
    B) Muscle weakness
    C) Loss of balance
    D) Double vision

3. What is the common cause of ischemic stroke?
    A) Hemorrhage
    B) Clot in the brain blood vessels
    C) Trauma to the head
    D) Tumor in the brain

4. A patient with Alzheimer's disease often exhibits which of the following symptoms?
    A) Memory loss
    B) Hyperactivity
    C) Hypertension
    D) Hypothermia

5. The Glasgow Coma Scale (GCS) is used to assess what?
    A) Heart rate
    B) Level of consciousness
    C) Blood pressure
    D) Blood glucose level

6. What is a primary treatment method for seizures in patients with epilepsy?
    A) Anticonvulsant medication
    B) Diuretics
    C) Antibiotics
    D) Beta-blockers

7. What condition is characterized by an abnormal accumulation of cerebrospinal fluid in the brain?
    A) Encephalitis
    B) Hydrocephalus
    C) Meningitis
    D) Glioblastoma

8. What is the primary symptom of myasthenia gravis?
    A) Muscle weakness
    B) Tremor
    C) Paralysis
    D) Hypotonia

9. Which of the following conditions can cause temporary paralysis and sensory disturbances?
    A) Stroke
    B) Transient ischemic attack (TIA)
    C) Parkinson's disease
    D) Epilepsy

10. Which part of the brain is primarily affected by Parkinson's disease?
    A) Frontal lobe
    B) Parietal lobe
    C) Substantia nigra
    D) Cerebellum

11. What is the most common type of headache?
    A) Migraine
    B) Cluster headache
    C) Tension-type headache
    D) Sinus headache

12. Which of the following is NOT a typical symptom of a brain tumour?
    A) Persistent headaches
    B) Seizures
    C) Changes in vision
    D) Hypertension

13. In which condition is a lumbar puncture most helpful for diagnosis?
    A) Multiple sclerosis
    B) Meningitis
    C) Parkinson's disease
    D) Alzheimer's disease

14. What is the primary role of dopamine in the brain?
    A) Regulate heart rate
    B) Regulate mood and motor control
    C) Regulate body temperature
    D) Regulate blood pressure

15. Which of the following disorders is characterized by excessive sleepiness during the day?
    A) Insomnia
    B) Sleep apnea
    C) Narcolepsy
    D) Sleepwalking

16. Which of the following is a common early Amyotrophic Lateral Sclerosis (ALS) symptom?
    A) Muscle weakness in hands, arms, or legs
    B) Tremors
    C) Double vision
    D) Slurred speech

17. Which type of stroke is characterized by bleeding within the brain?
    A) Ischemic stroke
    B) Hemorrhagic stroke
    C) Transient ischemic attack
    D) Embolic stroke

18. Which diagnostic tool is most often used to diagnose epilepsy?
    A) Computed Tomography (CT) scan
    B) Electroencephalogram (EEG)
    C) Magnetic Resonance Imaging (MRI)
    D) Positron Emission Tomography (PET) scan

Musculoskeletal Nursing

1. Which is the most common type of arthritis?
    A) Rheumatoid arthritis
    B) Osteoarthritis
    C) Gouty arthritis
    D) Septic arthritis

2. What is the most common initial treatment for a patient with a fracture?
    A) Amputation
    B) Immobilization
    C) Physical therapy
    D) Administration of pain medication

3. What is the term for a decrease in bone mass and density leading to an increased risk of fractures?
    A) Arthritis
    B) Tendonitis
    C) Osteoporosis
    D) Scoliosis

4. What is a common symptom of fibromyalgia?
    A) Widespread muscle pain and tenderness
    B) High fever
    C) Weight gain
    D) Hypertension

5. What is the primary concern for a patient with a hip fracture?
    A) Infection
    B) Mobility
    C) Pain control
    D) Weight loss

6. The deformity caused by the chronic inflammation in rheumatoid arthritis is due to?
    A) Bone loss
    B) Synovial membrane thickening
    C) Joint space narrowing
    D) All of the above

7. Scoliosis is a condition characterized by:
    A) Forward curvature of the spine
    B) Sideway curvature of the spine
    C) Backward curvature of the spine
    D) Inability to bend the spine

8. Carpal tunnel syndrome is commonly associated with:
    A) Prolonged typing or repetitive hand movements
    B) Overuse of the lower limbs
    C) Poor posture
    D) Excessive weight lifting

9. A sprain primarily affects which structure?
    A) Bone
    B) Muscle
    C) Ligament
    D) Tendon

10. Gout is a form of arthritis characterized by the following:
    A) The destruction of joint cartilage and underlying bone
    B) The deposition of uric acid crystals in the joint
    C) The overgrowth of bone spurs around the joint
    D) The inflammation and thickening of the synovial membrane

11. Which bone disorder is associated with vitamin D deficiency?
    A) Rickets
    B) Osteoporosis
    C) Paget's disease
    D) Osteoarthritis

12. A child with "growing pains" in the legs is likely experiencing:
    A) Osteomyelitis
    B) Rheumatoid arthritis
    C) Muscular dystrophy
    D) None of the above

13. The bone disease that is characterized by the excessive breakdown and formation of bone tissue is:
    A) Osteoporosis
    B) Paget's disease
    C) Rickets
    D) Arthritis

14. In a patient with a bone fracture, the healthcare provider should initially assess the following:
    A) Swelling
    B) Pain level
    C) Circulation, sensation, and motion (CSM)
    D) Bone deformity

15. A positive Phalen's test is indicative of which condition?
    A) Rheumatoid arthritis
    B) Carpal tunnel syndrome
    C) Gout
    D) Osteoarthritis

16. The most common type of joint replacement surgery is:
    A) Shoulder replacement
    B) Elbow replacement
    C) Knee replacement
    D) Hip replacement

17. What is the leading cause of musculoskeletal injuries in the elderly?
    A) Sports injuries
    B) Falls
    C) Car accidents
    D) Work-related injuries

18. The degeneration characterizes osteoarthritis:
    A) Muscles
    B) Ligaments
    C) Joint cartilage
    D) Tendons

Endocrine Nursing

1. Which hormone regulates blood sugar levels?
    A) Insulin
    B) Glucagon
    C) Both A and B
    D) Thyroxine

2. Which gland produces cortisol?
    A) Pancreas
    B) Thyroid
    C) Adrenal
    D) Pituitary

3. What is the primary treatment for hypothyroidism?
    A) Synthetic thyroxine
    B) Dietary changes
    C) Insulin administration
    D) Surgical removal of the thyroid

4. What is a common sign of hyperglycemia?
    A) Rapid weight gain
    B) Increased urination and thirst
    C) Chills and sweats
    D) Hypotension

5. Graves' disease is an autoimmune disorder that primarily affects which gland?
    A) Adrenal
    B) Thyroid
    C) Pancreas
    D) Parathyroid

6. Diabetic ketoacidosis (DKA) is a severe complication of which type of diabetes?
    A) Type 1
    B) Type 2
    C) Gestational diabetes
    D) All of the above

7. Which hormone is primarily responsible for regulating the body's metabolism?
    - **A)** Cortisol
    - **B)** Insulin
    - **C)** Thyroxine
    - **D)** Testosterone

8. A patient with Cushing's syndrome will likely exhibit which symptom?
    - **A)** Rapid weight loss
    - **B)** Moon face and buffalo hump
    - **C)** Hypotension
    - **D)** Hypoglycemia

9. Which disorder is characterized by the excessive production of growth hormones in adults?
    - **A)** Gigantism
    - **B)** Acromegaly
    - **C)** Dwarfism
    - **D)** Addison's disease

10. Addison's disease is primarily caused by the dysfunction of which gland?
    - **A)** Adrenal
    - **B)** Thyroid
    - **C)** Pancreas
    - **D)** Parathyroid

11. Which is a common symptom of hypoglycemia?
    - **A)** Increased urination
    - **B)** Tremors and sweating
    - **C)** Polydipsia
    - **D)** Weight gain

12. Which hormone is deficient in Addison's disease?
    - **A)** Cortisol
    - **B)** Thyroxine
    - **C)** Insulin
    - **D)** Glucagon

13. Which of the following is a common complication of diabetes?
    - **A)** Cardiovascular disease
    - **B)** Hypertension
    - **C)** Renal disease
    - **D)** All of the above

14. The hormone epinephrine is produced by which gland?
    - **A)** Adrenal
    - **B)** Thyroid
    - **C)** Pancreas
    - **D)** Pituitary

15. In Hashimoto's disease, which gland is affected?
    - **A)** Thyroid
    - **B)** Parathyroid
    - **C)** Adrenal
    - **D)** Pituitary

16. The primary function of parathyroid hormone is to:
    A) Regulate blood calcium levels
    B) Control metabolism
    C) Regulate blood sugar levels
    D) Control growth and development

17. Which hormone regulates the body's sleep-wake cycle?
    A) Melatonin
    B) Serotonin
    C) Dopamine
    D) Adrenaline

18. Diabetes insipidus is characterized by:
    A) Hypoglycemia
    B) Hyperglycemia
    C) Excessive thirst and urination
    D) Weight gain

Hematological and Immunological Nursing

1. What is the primary function of the red blood cells?
    A) Transport nutrients
    B) Carry oxygen
    C) Fight infection
    D) Aid in clotting

2. Which blood component aids in clotting?
    A) Red blood cells
    B) Platelets
    C) White blood cells
    D) Plasma

3. Which condition is characterized by a lower-than-normal count of red blood cells?
    A) Thrombocytopenia
    B) Leukemia
    C) Anemia
    D) Hemophilia

4. What is a common symptom of anaemia?
    A) Fatigue
    B) Fever
    C) Rapid heartbeat
    D) Both A and C

5. Which disorder is characterized by an overproduction of white blood cells?
    A) Anemia
    B) Leukemia
    C) Hemophilia
    D) Thrombocytopenia

6. What is the primary function of the white blood cells?
    A) Fight infection
    B) Carry oxygen
    C) Aid in clotting
    D) Transport nutrients

7. Which condition is characterized by an excessive number of platelets?
    A) Thrombocytosis
    B) Thrombocytopenia
    C) Anemia
    D) Leukemia

8. Which blood group is known as the universal donor?
    A) A
    B) B
    C) AB
    D) O

9. Which blood group is known as the universal recipient?
    A) A
    B) B
    C) AB
    D) O

10. A nurse is preparing to administer a blood transfusion. Which action is most important?
    A) Check the patient's vital signs
    B) Verify the blood type
    C) Infuse saline solution concurrently
    D) Both A and B

11. Which is a primary sign of an allergic reaction to a blood transfusion?
    A) Fever and chills
    B) Sudden drop in blood pressure
    C) Pale skin
    D) Increase in pulse rate

12. Sickle cell anaemia is characterized by which type of red blood cells?
    A) Oval-shaped
    B) Square-shaped
    C) Crescent-shaped
    D) Round-shaped

13. What is the most common type of leukaemia in adults?
    A) Acute Lymphoblastic Leukemia (ALL)
    B) Chronic Myeloid Leukemia (CML)
    C) Acute Myeloid Leukemia (AML)
    D) Chronic Lymphocytic Leukemia (CLL)

14. What is a common sign of deep vein thrombosis (DVT)?
    A) Swelling in one leg
    B) Chest pain
    C) Shortness of breath
    D) Both A and C

15. What type of medication is commonly administered to prevent clotting?
    A) Antibiotics
    B) Anticoagulants
    C) Analgesics
    D) Antivirals

16. What is the main characteristic of the autoimmune disorder lupus?
    A) Overactive immune response
    B) Weakened immune response
    C) Immune response to foreign substances
    D) No immune response

17. Which type of hepatitis is vaccine-preventable?
    A) Hepatitis A
    B) Hepatitis B
    C) Hepatitis C
    D) Both A and B

18. What is a common symptom of HIV/AIDS?
    A) Fever
    B) Fatigue
    C) Weight loss
    D) All of the above

19. What is the primary test to diagnose HIV?
    A) ELISA test
    B) Liver function test
    C) Blood count test
    D) All of the above

20. What is the primary treatment for HIV/AIDS?
    A) Antibiotics
    B) Antiretroviral therapy
    C) Analgesics
    D) Steroids

21. Hemophilia is a disorder characterized by:
    A) Excessive bleeding
    B) Excessive clotting
    C) Low platelet count
    D) High white blood cell count

22. Sepsis is a potentially life-threatening condition caused by:
    A) An overactive immune response
    B) A weakened immune response
    C) An immune response to a severe infection
    D) A complete lack of immune response

23. Which condition is characterized by an underactive immune system?
    A) Autoimmune disorder
    B) Allergy
    C) Immunodeficiency
    D) Hypersensitivity

24. Which medication is used to treat autoimmune diseases by suppressing the immune system?
- **A)** Antibiotics
- **B)** Analgesics
- **C)** Antivirals
- **D)** Immunosuppressants

ANSWER KEY

Cardiovascular Nursing

1. **C)** Atrial depolarization: The P wave represents atrial depolarization or the electrical conduction that triggers the atria to contract.
2. **A)** S1: S1 is the heart sound made by the closure of the mitral and tricuspid valves.
3. **C)** Bradycardia: Bradycardia, or a slow heart rate, is not typically a symptom of CHF. Instead, tachycardia is expected as the heart works harder to pump blood.
4. **B)** Vasodilator: Nitroglycerin is a vasodilator that relaxes (widens) blood vessels, improving blood flow and reducing the heart's workload.
5. **A)** At the 5th intercostal space at the left midclavicular line: This is the location of the apex of the heart where the apical pulse can be best palpated.
6. **C)** Blood Urea Nitrogen (BUN): BUN is typically used to assess kidney function, not heart disease risk.
7. **D)** Hypertension: A blood pressure reading of 150/95 mmHg would be classified as hypertension (high blood pressure).
8. **B)** Unstable angina: Unstable angina is characterized by unpredictable symptoms and may not be relieved by nitroglycerin or rest.
9. **D)** All of the above: All these are potential signs of digoxin toxicity and should be reported immediately.
10. **D)** Class IV: Class IV heart failure is the most severe and involves symptoms at rest.
11. **A)** Oxygen: Providing oxygen is typically the first intervention for a patient experiencing chest pain to increase oxygen supply to the heart muscle.
12. **B)** Monitoring the patient's vital signs closely: After cardiac catheterization, it's essential to monitor the patient's vital signs for any changes that may indicate complications.
13. **A)** Distant, muffled heart sounds: This can be a sign of a pericardial effusion in pericarditis, which can cause the heart sounds to be faint or distant.
14. **D)** Activated partial thromboplastin time (aPTT): The aPTT is used to monitor the effectiveness of heparin therapy.
15. **C)** Substernal, radiating, and lasting longer than 30 minutes: These are typical characteristics of pain associated with myocardial ischemia.
16. **C)** Pulmonary oedema: Left-sided heart failure can lead to fluid buildup in the lungs or pulmonary oedema.
17. **C)** High HDL cholesterol levels: High HDL cholesterol levels are protective against CAD, not a risk factor.
18. **B)** Ability to decrease heart rate and contractility: Beta-blockers are used in heart failure primarily for their ability to lower heart rate and contractility, reducing the heart's workload and oxygen demand.

Pulmonary Nursing

1. **D)** All of the above: All these symptoms are common in COPD as the disease primarily affects the airways and air sacs in the lungs.
2. **A)** Crackles: Crackles are a common breath sound heard in pneumonia due to fluid accumulation in the alveoli.
3. **C)** Lack of surfactant: In premature infants, RDS is often caused by a lack of surfactant, which helps keep the tiny air sacs in the lungs open.
4. **A)** Emphysema: Emphysema is characterized by the destruction of the alveolar walls, resulting in fewer, larger alveoli.
5. **B)** The amount of carbon dioxide in the blood: PaCO2 reflects the partial pressure of carbon dioxide in the blood, providing information about how well the lungs are removing this waste product.
6. **A)** Asthma: Asthma is characterized by an overreaction of the tracheobronchial tree to various stimuli, causing inflammation and narrowing of the airways.
7. **C)** Tuberculosis: The Mantoux test, or tuberculin skin test, is used to identify a tuberculosis infection.
8. **C)** Wheezing: Tuberculosis generally does not cause wheezing; symptoms typically include chest pain, a productive, sometimes bloody cough, and systemic symptoms like night sweats and weight loss.
9. **B)** Maintain a clear airway: While all these options are essential in care, the primary goal in treating pneumonia is maintaining a clear airway to ensure adequate oxygenation.
10. **B)** Smoking cigarettes: Cigarette smoking is the number one risk factor for lung cancer.
11. **B)** Diminished breath sounds on the affected side: Pleural effusion, or fluid buildup in the pleural space, can cause diminished breath sounds on the affected side due to the fluid blocking sound transmission.
12. **D)** All of the above: Pulmonary function tests measure the capacity and function of the lungs, can aid in diagnosing lung disease, and can help identify the cause of shortness of breath.
13. **B)** Decreased respiratory rate: An acute asthma exacerbation would typically result in an increased respiratory rate due to difficulty in breathing, not a decreased rate.
14. **C)** Begin oxygen therapy: Oxygen therapy is the immediate nursing intervention for a suspected pulmonary embolism to improve oxygenation.
15. **D)** Hypotension: A tension pneumothorax can lead to decreased venous return to the heart due to pressure on the vena cava, leading to hypotension.
16. **B)** Oxygen therapy: Oxygen therapy is the primary intervention for COPD to improve oxygenation.
17. **C)** Tachycardia: Theophylline can lead to tachycardia, or an increased heart rate, as a side effect.
18. **C)** Chronic hypoxia: Clubbing of the fingers is associated with chronic hypoxia, or low oxygen levels over a long period.

Gastrointestinal Nursing

1. **A)** Produce bile: The liver produces bile, essential for digestion and absorption of fats and fat-soluble vitamins in the small intestine.
2. **C)** Small intestine: While Crohn's disease can affect any part of the GI tract from the mouth to the anus, it most commonly affects the end of the small intestine (the ileum) and the beginning of the colon.
3. **C)** Diarrhea: GERD typically causes heartburn, chest pain, dyspepsia, and regurgitation, but not usually diarrhoea.
4. **D)** Popcorn and seeds: These small, hard particles can become lodged in the diverticula and lead to inflammation.
5. **A)** Helicobacter pylori infection: This bacterium is a common cause of peptic ulcers.
6. **C)** Obesity: Obesity is a risk factor for gallstones.
7. **B)** Fatty stools: 'Steatorrhea' refers to the excretion of abnormal quantities of fat in the faeces.
8. **C)** Gluten: Individuals with celiac disease must avoid foods containing gluten, a protein found in wheat, barley, and rye.
9. **C)** Inguinal hernia: Inguinal hernias are the most common type in both genders.
10. **A)** Right lower quadrant pain: Appendicitis typically presents with pain in the right lower quadrant of the abdomen.
11. **A)** High-fiber diet: A high-fibre diet is typically the first-line treatment for haemorrhoids, helping to soften the stool and reduce strain during bowel movements.
12. **A)** Hepatitis: Jaundice, a yellowing of the skin and eyes due to elevated bilirubin levels in the blood, is a common symptom of liver diseases such as hepatitis.
13. **A)** Peptic ulcer disease: "Coffee-ground" vomitus, or vomit that looks like coffee grounds, is often a sign of bleeding in the stomach, which is commonly caused by peptic ulcer disease.
14. **C)** Decompression: In the postoperative period, a nasogastric tube is typically used for decompression to remove gas and fluids and prevent abdominal distension.
15. **D)** Excessive exercise: While physical activity promotes healthy bowel function, excessive practice does not typically cause constipation. The other options (inadequate fluid intake, inadequate fibre intake, and overuse of laxatives) can all contribute to constipation.
16. **B)** Ascites: Ascites, the accumulation of fluid in the peritoneal cavity, is a common complication of cirrhosis.
17. **B)** Increased amylase levels: In pancreatitis, enzymes such as amylase and lipase become elevated as the pancreas is inflamed, and the cells release these enzymes into the bloodstream.
18. **D)** Cirrhosis: Esophageal varices are dilated veins in the oesophagus that can rupture and bleed and are a common complication of cirrhosis.

Renal and Urinary Nursing

1. **A)** Hematuria: Hematuria, or blood in the urine, is a common sign of a urinary tract infection.
2. **C)** Production of insulin: The pancreas, not the kidneys, is responsible for insulin production.
3. **C)** Kidneys: Pyelonephritis is an infection of the kidneys, often resulting from a urinary tract infection that has moved up the urinary system.
4. **A)** Dehydration: Dehydration is a significant risk factor for developing kidney stones.
5. **B)** Proteinuria: Proteinuria, or high protein levels in the urine, is a crucial symptom of glomerulonephritis.
6. **C)** Long-standing disease: Chronic renal failure is a long-standing disease and refers to the gradual loss of kidney function over time.
7. **B)** To remove urine from the bladder: A urinary catheter drains urine from the bladder when a person cannot urinate independently.
8. **B)** A condition where multiple cysts develop in the kidneys: Polycystic kidney disease is a genetic disorder characterized by the growth of numerous cysts filled with fluid in the kidneys.
9. **C)** To filter toxins and waste from the blood: The primary function of dialysis in a patient with kidney failure is to perform the kidneys' filtering function - removing waste, salt, and extra water to prevent them from building up in the body.
10. **B)** Kidney transplant: A patient with end-stage renal disease (ESR**D)** may require a kidney transplant as part of their treatment.
11. **A)** Hematuria: Blood in the urine, or hematuria, is a common symptom of bladder cancer.
12. **A)** Overactive bladder: An overactive bladder, often resulting in a frequent urge to urinate, is a common cause of urinary incontinence in older adults.
13. **A)** Low-sodium, low-protein diet: A diet low in sodium and protein can help control symptoms of chronic kidney disease and delay progression.
14. **B)** Angiotensin-converting enzyme (ACE) inhibitors: ACE inhibitors often decrease proteinuria in patients with nephrotic syndrome.
15. **A)** Decreased creatinine clearance: Decreased creatinine clearance can indicate reduced kidney function as kidneys are not efficiently removing creatinine from the blood.
16. **A)** Kidney stones: Hydronephrosis, or the swelling of a kidney due to a buildup of urine, can be caused by underlying conditions such as kidney stones that block the normal flow of urine.
17. **A)** Anuria, or the absence of urine production, can be an early sign of acute kidney injury.
18. **B)** Urge incontinence: Urge incontinence is caused by an overactive detrusor muscle, which leads to a sudden and powerful need to urinate.

Neurological Nursing

1. **C)** Bradycardia: Bradycardia is not a classic sign of Parkinson's disease. The primary symptoms are tremors, rigidity, and postural instability.
2. **A)** Fatigue: Fatigue is often the primary initial symptom in patients with multiple sclerosis.
3. **B)** Clot in the brain blood vessels: Ischemic stroke is most often caused by a clot blocking blood flow in the brain.
4. **A)** Memory loss: Memory loss is a common symptom of Alzheimer's disease.
5. **B)** Level of consciousness: The Glasgow Coma Scale is used to assess a patient's level of consciousness after a brain injury.
6. **A)** Anticonvulsant medication: Anticonvulsant medications are the primary treatment for seizures in patients with epilepsy.
7. **B)** Hydrocephalus: Hydrocephalus is characterized by an abnormal accumulation of cerebrospinal fluid in the brain.
8. **A)** Muscle weakness: The primary symptom of myasthenia gravis is muscle weakness.
9. **B)** Transient ischemic attack (TIA): A TIA, often called a mini-stroke, can cause temporary paralysis and sensory disturbances.
10. **C)** Substantia nigra: Parkinson's disease primarily affects the substantia nigra, a part of the brain that plays a vital role in reward and movement.
11. **C)** Tension-type headache: Tension-type headaches are the most common.
12. **D)** Hypertension: Hypertension is not a typical symptom of a brain tumour. Persistent headaches, seizures, and vision changes are common symptoms.
13. **B)** Meningitis: A lumbar puncture, where a needle is inserted into the spinal canal to collect cerebrospinal fluid, is most helpful for diagnosing conditions like meningitis.
14. **B)** Regulate mood and motor control: Dopamine primarily helps regulate mood and motor control in the brain.
15. **C)** Narcolepsy: Narcolepsy is characterized by excessive daytime sleepiness, often with episodes of falling asleep suddenly.
16. **A)** Muscle weakness in hands, arms, or legs: Muscle weakness in these areas is often an early symptom of ALS.
17. **B)** Hemorrhagic stroke: Hemorrhagic stroke is characterized by bleeding within the brain.
18. **B)** Electroencephalogram (EEG): An EEG, which measures electrical activity in the brain, is the most commonly used tool to diagnose epilepsy.

Musculoskeletal Nursing

1. **B)** Osteoarthritis: This is the most common form of arthritis, typically affecting older individuals and resulting from wear and tear on the joints over time.
2. **B)** Immobilization: This is often the first step in treating a fracture to prevent further damage and allow the bone to begin healing.
3. **C)** Osteoporosis: This condition involves decreased bone mass and density, increasing the risk of fractures.
4. **A)** Widespread muscle pain and tenderness: These are common symptoms of fibromyalgia, a chronic condition affecting the musculoskeletal system.
5. **B)** Mobility: A hip fracture can significantly impact a patient's mobility, often requiring surgery and extensive rehabilitation.
6. **D)** All of the above: Chronic inflammation in rheumatoid arthritis leads to bone loss, synovial membrane thickening, and joint space narrowing, contributing to deformity.
7. **B)** Sideways curvature of the spine: Scoliosis involves a sideways curvature that usually occurs during the growth spurt before puberty.
8. **A)** Prolonged typing or repetitive hand movements: These activities can pressure the median nerve, leading to carpal tunnel syndrome.
9. **C)** Ligament: Sprains occur when a ligament (the tissue that connects two bones) is stretched or torn.
10. **B)** The deposition of uric acid crystals in the joint: Gout involves the buildup of uric acid crystals in a joint, causing inflammation and severe pain.
11. **A)** Rickets: This condition is caused by a deficiency of vitamin D, calcium, or phosphate, leading to soft and weak bones in children.
12. **D)** None of the above: Growing pains are joint in children and are often not linked to severe conditions. They typically resolve on their own.
13. **B)** Paget's disease: This bone disorder involves the excessive breakdown and reconstruction of bone tissue, leading to weakened and deformed bones.
14. **C)** Circulation, sensation, and motion (CSM): This is the initial assessment for a patient with a fracture to ensure no damage to the nerves or blood vessels.
15. **B)** Carpal tunnel syndrome: A positive Phalen's test (flexing the wrists for a minute) can suggest carpal tunnel syndrome, a condition that affects the nerves in the hand.
16. **C)** Knee replacement: This is the most common joint replacement surgery, often performed when arthritis or injury severely damages the knee joint.
17. **B)** Falls: Falls are the leading cause of musculoskeletal injuries in the elderly, often resulting in fractures and other damages.
18. **C)** Joint cartilage: Osteoarthritis involves the degeneration of joint cartilage, the protective tissue at the ends of bones that allows smooth movement of joints.

Endocrine Nursing

1. **C)** Both A and B: Insulin and glucagon work together to regulate blood sugar levels.
2. **C)** Adrenal: The adrenal glands produce cortisol, a steroid hormone that helps the body respond to stress.
3. **A)** Synthetic thyroxine: Hypothyroidism is commonly treated with synthetic thyroxine (T4), a hormone usually produced by the thyroid gland.
4. **B)** Increased urination and thirst: Hyperglycemia, or high blood sugar, often causes increased urination and thirst.
5. **B)** Thyroid: Graves' disease is an autoimmune disorder that causes the thyroid gland to produce excessive amounts of thyroid hormone.
6. **A)** Type 1: Diabetic ketoacidosis (DKA) is a severe complication commonly associated with Type 1 diabetes.
7. **C)** Thyroxine: Thyroxine, produced by the thyroid gland, is primarily responsible for regulating the body's metabolism.
8. **B)** Moon face and buffalo hump: These are characteristic symptoms of Cushing's syndrome, caused by an excessive cortisol level in the body.
9. **B)** Acromegaly: Acromegaly is a disorder characterized by excessive growth hormone production in adults, leading to enlarged extremities and facial features.
10. **A)** Adrenal: Addison's disease is caused by the failure of the adrenal glands to produce sufficient amounts of cortisol and aldosterone.
11. **B)** Tremors and sweating are common symptoms of hypoglycemia or low blood sugar.
12. **A)** Cortisol: Addison's disease is characterized by a deficiency of cortisol, a hormone produced by the adrenal glands.
13. **D)** All of the above: Diabetes can lead to various complications, including cardiovascular disease, hypertension, and renal disease.
14. **A)** Adrenal: The adrenal glands produce epinephrine, also known as adrenaline, which prepares the body for a 'fight or flight' response.
15. **A)** Thyroid: Hashimoto's disease is an autoimmune disorder that primarily affects the thyroid gland, leading to hypothyroidism.
16. **A)** Regulate blood calcium levels: Parathyroid hormone is crucial for regulating the amount of calcium in the blood and bones.
17. **A)** Melatonin: Melatonin, produced by the pineal gland, is the hormone responsible for regulating the body's sleep-wake cycle.
18. **C)** Excessive thirst and urination: Diabetes insipidus is characterized by extreme thirst and excessive urination due to the kidney's impaired ability to concentrate urine.

Hematological and Immunological Nursing

1. **B)** Carry oxygen. The primary function of red blood cells is to carry oxygen to body tissues.
2. **B)** Platelets. Platelets aid in clotting to prevent excessive bleeding.
3. **C)** Anemia. A low count of red blood cells characterizes anaemia.
4. **D)** A low red blood cell count characterizes A and C. Anemia.
5. **B)** Leukemia. Fatigue and a rapid heartbeat are common symptoms of anaemia.
6. **A)** Fight infection. Leukaemia is a type of cancer characterized by the overproduction of white blood cells.
7. **A)** Thrombocytosis. The primary function of white blood cells is to fight infection.
8. **D)** O. Blood group O can donate to all other blood groups. Hence it's known as the universal donor.
9. **C)** AB. Blood group AB can receive from all other blood groups. Hence it's known as the universal recipient.
10. **D)** Both A and B. Before administering a blood transfusion, checking the patient's vital signs and verifying the blood type is crucial.
11. **A)** Fever and chills. Fever and chills are primary signs of an allergic reaction to a blood transfusion.
12. **C)** Crescent-shaped. In sickle cell anaemia, red blood cells are crescent or sickle-shaped.
13. **D)** Chronic Lymphocytic Leukemia (CLL). Chronic Lymphocytic Leukemia (CLL) is adults' most common type of leukaemia.
14. **A)** Swelling in one leg. Swelling in one leg is a common sign of deep vein thrombosis (DVT).
15. **B)** Anticoagulants. Anticoagulants are commonly administered to prevent clotting.
16. **A)** Overactive immune response. Lupus is an autoimmune disorder characterized by an overactive immune response.
17. **D)** Both A and B. Vaccines are available for Hepatitis A and B.
18. **D)** All of the above. Fever, fatigue, and weight loss are common symptoms of HIV/AIDS.
19. **A)** ELISA test. The ELISA test is primarily used to diagnose HIV.
20. **B)** Antiretroviral therapy. Antiretroviral therapy is the primary treatment for HIV/AIDS.
21. **A)** Excessive bleeding. Hemophilia is a disorder characterized by excessive bleeding.
22. **C)** An immune response to a severe infection. An immune response to a severe disease causes sepsis.
23. **C)** Immunodeficiency. An underactive immune system characterizes immunodeficiency.
24. **D)** Immunosuppressants. Immunosuppressants are used to treat autoimmune diseases by suppressing the immune system.

FAQS PART 1

What is the CMSRN exam?
The CMSRN (Certified Medical-Surgical Registered Nurse) exam is a certification examination that validates a nurse's knowledge and skills in medical-surgical nursing.

Who administers the CMSRN exam?
The CMSRN exam is administered by the Medical-Surgical Nursing Certification Board (MSNCB).

Who can take the CMSRN exam?
Registered Nurses with at least two years of experience in medical-surgical nursing and a minimum of 2000 hours of practice within the past three years are eligible to take the CMSRN exam.

What is the format of the CMSRN exam?
The CMSRN exam is a computer-based test consisting of 150 multiple-choice questions.

How long is the CMSRN exam?
Test-takers are given 3 hours to complete the CMSRN exam.

What subjects are covered on the CMSRN exam?
The CMSRN exam covers various topics, including pulmonary, cardiac, gastrointestinal, urinary, neurological, musculoskeletal, and endocrine systems, and professional issues like patient education and nursing management.

What score is needed to pass the CMSRN exam?
A panel of experts determines the passing score for the CMSRN exam, which varies based on the difficulty of the test.

How can I prepare for the CMSRN exam?
Preparation for the CMSRN exam can include studying textbooks, attending review courses, and taking practice tests.

How often can I take the CMSRN exam?
If you do not pass the CMSRN exam, you may reapply and retake the exam after a 90-day waiting.

How much does the CMSRN exam cost?
The CMSRN exam costs $375 for non-members of the Academy of Medical-Surgical Nurses (AMSN) and $255 for members.

Is the CMSRN certification worth it?
Earning CMSRN certification can demonstrate your commitment to professional growth, enhance your credibility, and open up opportunities for advancement in medical-surgical nursing.

What happens if I fail the CMSRN exam?
If you fail the CMSRN exam, you can reapply and retake the test after a 90-day waiting period.

How often do I need to recertify?
CMSRN certification is valid for five years, after which you must recertify by demonstrating ongoing professional development or retaking the exam.

Can I reschedule the CMSRN exam?
Yes, you can reschedule the exam. However, a fee may be associated with rescheduling, depending on the timing of the change.

What is the best way to study for the CMSRN exam?
The best way to study varies by individual. Some find review courses helpful, while others prefer independent study with textbooks and practice tests.

How many nurses are CMSRN certified?
As of my knowledge, cut-off in September 2021, more than 30,000 nurses worldwide have achieved CMSRN certification. Please check the MSNCB's official website for updated statistics.

What are the benefits of being CMSRN certified?
CMSRN certification validates your expertise in medical-surgical nursing, can make you more competitive in the job market, and may lead to higher compensation.

What resources are available to prepare for the CMSRN exam?
Resources available include the MSNCB's official CMSRN examination review book, online practice tests, review courses, and study groups.

Do employers value the CMSRN certification?
Many employers value the CMSRN certification as it demonstrates a nurse's commitment to excellence and ongoing professional development.

Does the CMSRN exam require renewal?
Yes, the CMSRN certification requires renewal every five years through professional development or re-examination.

How is hypertension managed in a patient?
Hypertension management is a combination of lifestyle modifications and medication. Lifestyle changes may include reducing salt and alcohol intake, regular exercise, maintaining a healthy weight, and quitting smoking. If these changes aren't enough, medications such as ACE inhibitors, angiotensin II receptor blockers, calcium channel blockers, and diuretics might be introduced. Nurses play a vital role in patient education, ensuring compliance with treatment, and regularly monitoring blood pressure.

What's involved in the care of a patient post-cardiac surgery?
Post-cardiac surgery care is multifaceted. It includes pain management, monitoring for signs of complications like infection or arrhythmias, managing wound care, and ensuring optimal respiratory function. Rehabilitation also begins early, with simple mobility exercises initially. Educating the patient and family on signs of complications, medication regimen, and lifestyle modifications is also essential.

What are key considerations in the care of a patient with a stroke?
Stroke care focuses on immediate stabilization, symptom management, and prevention of complications. Nurses must closely monitor vital signs and neurologic status and administer medications like tissue plasminogen activator (tPA) in ischemic stroke. Once the patient is stable, early mobilization, swallowing assessment, and speech therapy are initiated. Patient and family education about the disease, treatment regimen, and lifestyle changes is also vital.

How is diabetes managed in a patient?
Diabetes management involves a comprehensive approach. It includes maintaining blood glucose levels through dietary modifications, exercise, and medications or insulin as needed. Regular blood glucose and hemoglobin A1C monitoring is required to evaluate treatment effectiveness. Nurses play a crucial role in teaching patients self-monitoring techniques, medication management, foot care, and recognizing symptoms of hypo and hyperglycemia.

What are some treatments for breast cancer?
Breast cancer treatments are individualized based on the type, stage, and patient's health status. They may include surgery (lumpectomy, mastectomy), radiation therapy, chemotherapy, hormone therapy, and targeted therapies. Nurses must manage the side effects of these treatments, provide emotional support, educate patients on self-care, and coordinate care between different healthcare professionals.

How are pressure ulcers managed in nursing care?
Pressure ulcer management involves regular repositioning of the patient to offload pressure, maintaining skin hygiene, using pressure-relief devices, and appropriate wound dressings or debridement if necessary. Nutritional support for wound healing is also crucial. Nurses must assess the ulcer regularly for signs of infection and educate the patient and caregivers about prevention strategies.

What does a nurse do if a patient's oxygen saturation drops?
If a patient's oxygen saturation drops, the nurse should first ensure their airway is open and they are breathing adequately. The nurse might need to reposition the patient, increase the oxygen flow rate (if already on supplemental oxygen), or start oxygen therapy. Prompt notification to the healthcare provider is necessary for further assessment and interventions.

How does a nurse manage a patient's pain post-fracture?
Post-fracture pain management includes administering prescribed analgesics on schedule and evaluating their effectiveness. Non-pharmacological methods like positioning, distraction, relaxation techniques, and cold or heat application may also help. The nurse needs to regularly assess the patient's pain level, monitor for signs of complications, and educate the patient about the safe use of pain medication.

What dietary advice is given to a patient with liver cirrhosis?
In liver cirrhosis, the diet should be high in calories and protein to counteract malnutrition, but sodium intake should be limited to prevent fluid accumulation. Depending on the severity, certain nutrients might be restricted or supplemented. Nurses educate patients about suitable food choices, monitor their nutritional status, and coordinate with dietitians for individualized meal planning.

How are asthma attacks prevented in a patient?
Asthma attacks are prevented by controlling inflammation and avoiding triggers. This might involve the regular use of inhaled corticosteroids and long-acting bronchodilators alongside quick-relief medications for acute symptoms. Nurses educate patients on correct inhaler techniques, developing an asthma action plan, recognizing early signs of an exacerbation, and when to seek medical help.

How does a nurse care for a patient with thyroid disorders?
Care for patients with thyroid disorders includes administering medications such as levothyroxine or antithyroid drugs for hypothyroidism. Regular monitoring of vital signs, thyroid hormone levels, and the patient's response to treatment is essential. Nurses also educate patients about medication adherence, routine follow-up visits, and symptom management.

What nursing care is given to a patient with kidney disease?
Nursing care for kidney disease patients focuses on managing symptoms, preventing complications, and slowing disease progression. This could involve administering medications, dietary modifications, fluid management, and supporting dialysis or transplant procedures if needed. Nurses monitor the patient's vital signs, lab values, and fluid status and educate them about disease management.

What are the complications of chemotherapy in a cancer patient?
Chemotherapy can lead to various side effects, including nausea, vomiting, hair loss, fatigue, and mouth sores. More severe complications can include neutropenia leading to infections, anemia, thrombocytopenia causing easy bleeding, and neuropathy. Nurses are crucial in managing these side effects, educating patients, and coordinating care among the healthcare team.

How are burns managed in a patient?
Burn management includes pain control, preventing infection, promoting healing, and providing nutritional support. Initial care involves cooling the burn, cleaning with mild soap and water, and applying suitable dressings. For severe burns, fluid resuscitation, wound debridement, and possibly skin grafts might be required. Nurses closely monitor the patient's vital signs, wound healing, and psychological well-being.

How are COPD patients managed in nursing care?
COPD management relieves symptoms, prevents exacerbations, and improves overall health. This can include bronchodilator medications, oxygen therapy, pulmonary rehabilitation, and lifestyle modifications

like smoking cessation. Nurses educate patients about disease management, breathing exercises, and using drugs and oxygen. They also coordinate care among the healthcare team.

What are the critical aspects of care for a patient with heart failure?
Heart failure management involves medications to improve heart function, fluid management to prevent overload, monitoring for signs of worsening heart failure, and patient education. Nurses play a crucial role in administering and monitoring the effects of medications, assessing fluid status, and educating patients about self-care, including diet, exercise, and medication compliance.

How does a nurse manage a patient with a neurological disorder like Parkinson's?
Nursing care for Parkinson's disease focuses on maintaining mobility, promoting safe self-care, managing medications, and providing psychosocial support. Nurses help patients manage their medications, monitor for side effects, and coordinate with physical therapists for mobility training. They also provide education on the disease and support the patient's emotional well-being.

What are the nursing considerations for a patient with severe malnutrition?
For a patient with severe malnutrition, the nurse would administer nutritional supplementation as ordered, monitor the patient's vital signs and laboratory values, and observe for symptoms of refeeding syndrome. Education about a balanced diet and portion control is also essential. The nurse also coordinates with the dietitian for a tailored nutrition plan and monitors the patient's progress toward their nutritional goals.

What is the nurse's role in managing a patient with sepsis?
In sepsis management, nurses administer antibiotics and fluids as ordered, closely monitor vital signs, laboratory results, and organ function, and provide supportive care to alleviate symptoms. Early recognition of the deteriorating condition and prompt communication with the healthcare team is essential. Nurses also educate the patient and family about the condition and care plan.

How is a patient prepared for a surgical procedure?
Preparing a patient for surgery involves a preoperative assessment to identify potential risks, education about the procedure and recovery process, and physical preparation like fasting or skin cleansing. Nurses also provide emotional support, administer preoperative medications as ordered, and complete relevant documentation.

What are the nursing considerations for a patient undergoing radiation therapy?
Nursing considerations for patients undergoing radiation therapy include monitoring for side effects like skin reactions, fatigue, and altered taste. Nurses should provide skin care instructions, promote energy-conserving activities, and encourage dietary changes to combat taste changes. Emotional support and education about the therapy and its potential side effects are also crucial.

How does a nurse manage a patient with dementia?
Nursing management for dementia involves supporting cognitive function, ensuring a safe environment, managing behavioral changes, and providing psychosocial support. Nurses help with memory aids, establish routines to orient the patient, manage medications, and provide emotional support to patients and their families. They also coordinate with other healthcare professionals for a comprehensive care approach.

What is involved in the nursing care of a patient with anemia?
Anemia care involves treating the underlying cause, providing dietary education about iron-rich foods, administering prescribed medications or blood transfusions, and managing symptoms. Nurses monitor the patient's hemoglobin levels, vital signs, and response to treatment and educate the patient about managing fatigue and when to seek medical attention.

How does a nurse manage a patient with pneumonia?
Pneumonia management includes administration of antibiotics, oxygen therapy if needed, promoting hydration, and encouraging mobilization to clear lung secretions. Nurses monitor respiratory status, vital signs, and response to treatment. Nursing responsibilities include education about medication use, coughing techniques, and the importance of follow-up care.

What does wound care involve in nursing practice?
Wound care involves cleaning the wound, applying appropriate dressings, monitoring for signs of infection, and managing pain. Wound healing is promoted through nutritional support and mobilization as tolerated. Nurses also educate the patient and caregivers about wound care at home and when to report potential complications.

How does a nurse manage a patient in pain?
Pain management includes administering prescribed analgesics, assessing their effectiveness, and employing non-pharmacological methods such as relaxation techniques, heat or cold application, and distraction. Regularly reassessing the patient's pain and adjusting the pain management plan as needed is essential. Nurses also educate patients about the safe use of analgesics and side effects to monitor.

How is patient education conducted in nursing practice?
Patient education involves assessing their learning needs, readiness, and learning style, providing tailored information about their condition, treatment, self-care, and follow-up. Nurses use clear, simple language, provide written materials, and verify understanding through the teach-back method. Reinforcement and revision of education at different points in care are also necessary.

How does a nurse manage a patient with depression?
Managing a patient with depression involves providing a safe, supportive environment, administering prescribed antidepressants, and monitoring their effectiveness and potential side effects. Nurses also promote self-care activities and therapeutic communication to encourage expressing feelings and facilitate psychotherapy referrals. Patient and family education about the illness, treatment plan, and strategies to manage stress are also part of the nurse's role.

How does a nurse manage a patient with urinary incontinence?
Management of urinary incontinence includes interventions such as bladder training, scheduled toileting, and lifestyle modifications like fluid management. Nurses assist with the use of continence aids, administer medications if prescribed, and educate patients about pelvic floor exercises. They also provide emotional support and encourage patients to participate in social activities without embarrassment.

What are the nursing considerations for a patient with osteoporosis?
Nursing care for osteoporosis focuses on promoting bone health, preventing falls, managing pain, and facilitating mobility. Nurses administer prescribed medications, and provide education about weight-bearing exercises, dietary sources of calcium and vitamin D, and fall prevention strategies. They also assess the patient's pain level and monitor for complications like fractures.

How does a nurse care for a patient with a pressure ulcer?
Pressure ulcer care includes pressure relief, wound cleaning, application of appropriate dressings, and pain management. Nurses closely monitor the ulcer for signs of healing or infection and provide nutritional support for wound healing. Education about repositioning, skincare, and symptoms of illness is provided to the patient and caregivers.

How is a patient with sleep apnea managed in nursing care?
In managing sleep apnea, nurses might assist with using continuous positive airway pressure (CPAP) therapy, provide education about lifestyle changes like weight loss and smoking cessation, and monitor the patient for complications. They also coordinate care with other healthcare professionals and provide support and education to the patient and family about the disorder.

What are the nursing considerations for a patient with a pacemaker?
Nursing care for patients with pacemakers includes monitoring heart rhythm, assessing the pacemaker site for signs of infection, managing symptoms related to the heart's rate and rhythm, and providing patient education. Nurses teach patients about activity restrictions, symptom recognition, follow-up care, and the importance of carrying pacemaker identification information.

How does a nurse manage a patient with acute kidney injury?

Management of acute kidney injury involves monitoring renal function, fluid balance, and electrolyte levels, managing symptoms, and providing supportive care. Nurses administer prescribed medications, watch for complications, and educate patients about dietary modifications, medication use, and follow-up care. They also coordinate care with the nephrology team.

What is the role of a nurse in managing a patient with a drug overdose?
In a drug overdose, nurses provide supportive care, administer antidotes, closely monitor vital signs, neurologic status, and organ function, and prepare for potential emergency interventions. They also offer psychological support, assess for suicide risk if the overdose was intentional, and might refer the patient to substance abuse counseling.

How is a patient with alcohol withdrawal syndrome managed in nursing care?
Alcohol withdrawal management includes administering medications to reduce withdrawal symptoms, providing a safe and quiet environment, and close monitoring for signs of delirium tremens. Nurses also provide emotional support, engage the patient in substance abuse therapy, and provide education about the dangers of alcohol misuse and the benefits of sobriety.

What are nursing considerations for a patient receiving a blood transfusion?
During a blood transfusion, nurses monitor the patient closely for signs of transfusion reactions like fever, chills, rash, or difficulty breathing. They also ensure the correct blood product is given to the right patient, maintain intravenous access, and monitor vital signs before, during, and after the transfusion. Patient education about potential reactions and the need to report any discomfort is also critical.

How does a nurse manage a deep vein thrombosis (DVT) patient?
In managing DVT, nurses administer anticoagulant medications as prescribed, monitor for signs of improvement or complications like pulmonary embolism, and provide education about the condition. They also promote measures to prevent DVT, such as mobility, hydration, and compression stockings. Patient education about medication use, follow-up care, and lifestyle modifications is also part of the nurse's role.

FAQS PART 2

Question: How can a nurse deal with a depressed patient?
Answer: Mental status assessment, working with a psychiatrist, administration of psychotropic medication, counseling, relaxation techniques, and social support are also critical components of nursing care for a depressed patient. It may include medication administration and counseling support in the care plan. It is equally essential that the patient be educated concerning coping mechanisms, available treatment options, and the need for attending to follow-up appointments.

Question: What should a nurse do regarding a patient with urinary incontinence?
Answer: A nurse will assess the patient's problem based on its underlying cause, implement pelvic floor exercises, and teach the patient how to do bladder training, among other things. This may include incontinence products, as well as some types of behavioral intervention strategies. Patients should be educated on lifestyle changes, fluid management, and follow-up.

Question: How should a nurse manage osteoporosis?
Answer: Nursing concerns consist of fracture risk assessment, encouraging the intake of calcium and vitamin D, and implementation of measures aimed at reducing the occurrences of falls in patients with osteoporosis disease. Two critical aspects include weight-bearing exercises and adhering to medicine. Educating patients on bone health, its protection, and the need for continued follow-up is essential.

Question: What is entailed in caring for a patient with a pressure ulcer?
Answer: The nursing care of a pressure ulcer patient entails frequent checks, wound cleanings, and dressing changes. Promoting wound healing, offloading pressure from wounds, and improving the diet for faster recovery. Prevention and management are associated with patient education for skin care, positioning, and follow-up.

Question: Describe and evaluate ways of managing a patient with sleep apnea in nursing care.
Answer: A patient on sleep apnea nursing care entails CPAP therapy, weight control, and positioning therapy. It is, therefore, vital that appropriate education is provided on the correct utilization of CPAP machines, lifestyle changes, and why they are essential and should be done periodically.

Question: Describe Nursing considerations in a patient having a pacemaker.
Answer: Patient nursing considerations like monitoring the device function, looking for complications, and ensuring education. A cardiologist should be seen frequently. Patients must be educated about indicators of device failure and necessary lifestyle changes.

Question: What is the ideal way for a nurse to manage the situation with PKD?
Answer: Nursing care for patients with PKD includes managing pain, watching out for complications, and supporting renal functions. Patients should collaborate with genetic specialists for counseling and disease progression. Patients must be educated about symptom management, lifestyle changes, and routine follow-ups.

Question: How is glomerulonephritis managed through interventions?
Answer: Glomerulonephritis is followed by interventions including monitoring of renal functions, administration of anti-inflammatory agents, and symptom management. These include fluid and electrolyte balance, as well as blood pressure control. Educate about medication adherence, diet changes, and follow-up plans.

Question: What roles do nurses play in managing nephrotic syndrome?
Answer: Proteinuria control, management of edema, and prevention of complications are among nephrotic syndrome management components. Doctors can prescribe medications such as diuretics and immunosuppressant. The patient should be educated about medication adherence, dietary restrictions, and self-monitoring, which are vital for management success.

Question: How should hydro nephrosis be treated?
Answer: Hydro nephrosis treatment focuses on discovering the primary pathology and restoring renal filtration and excretion ability. This can involve the application of drugs, drainage procedures, surgery, or any other intervention that is deemed necessary. Such patient education teaches them to recognize symptoms, practice preventive approaches, and follow up.

Question: What is done for RCC?
Answer: Surgical resection of tumors, targeted therapies, and immunotherapies are interventions for RCC. Care of nursing includes monitoring complications while supporting recovery. It is essential to educate patients on postoperative care, the possible side effects that can arise from the treatment, and the need for follow-up.

Question: What nursing care interventions are required for kids with kidney stones?
Answer: Pain control, adequate hydration, and close follow-up are paramount components of nursing care for children with stone disease. Such interventions can involve nutritional modifications or medical prescriptions. Patients must be educated on preventive methods, diets, and the necessity of follow-up.

Question: What is the process of a Nurse dealing with nephrotic syndrome in a patient?
Answer: The management of nephrotic syndromes aims to reduce proteinuria, edema, and the development of complications. Examples of drugs are diuretics and immunosuppressants. Effective patient education on medication adherence, dietary restrictions, and self-monitoring are vital for improved diabetes management.

Question: How should hydro nephrosis be addressed when it comes to nursing care?
Answer: Achieving hydro nephrosis is based on etiology, obstruction release, and improving renal function. This could involve the use of medicines through drainage or performing surgical operations. Patients should be engaged in their learning process of symptom identification, prevention, and post-care.

Question: How do renal cell carcinoma interventions feature in nursing practice?
Answer: Surgical extirpation of the tumor, as well as targeted therapy with an anti-angiogenic drug and immunotherapy, are part of the interventions used to address RCC. Monitoring for complications and providing recovery support is part of nursing care. Educating patients on postoperative care, possible adverse effects of treatment, and the relevance of follow-up is necessary.

Question: What does one do to a patient during follow-up after a stroke attack?
Answer: Monitoring vital signs and assessing neurological status as interventional measures against possible complications in nursing care following a stroke. Physical therapy, speech therapy, occupational therapy, and rehabilitation strategies are vital. Patients must be educated about stroke recovery, taking their medications, and adhering to lifestyle changes.

Question: What do nurses apply under the management of epilepsy?
Answer: Nursing care for epilepsy includes giving out antiepileptic drugs, tracking the state of seizures, and teaching patients about medication use and seizure triggers. It is essential to work with health care providers in medicine adjustments and regularly control them. There is a need to educate patients about lifestyle changes & recognizing warning signs.

Question: Describe Neurodegenerative Disease and Nursing Care.
Answer: Symptom control, assistance with ADLs, and complication monitoring are the hallmarks of neurodegenerative disease nursing care. Working together with a multi-professional healthcare team on medication and intervention is essential. Patient education must cover the course of the disease, self-care techniques, and what kind of help exists.

Question: What can a nurse do for a patient with amyotrophic lateral sclerosis (ALS)?
Answer: However, caring for persons with ALS includes helping them with their daily needs, symptom management, and working together with healthcare professionals on interventions. They also have palliative care as well as emotional support. Education of patients about how the disease progresses, adaptive techniques and the support services that exist are imperative.

Question: What is the treatment plan for Guillain-Barre Syndrome in nursing care?
Answer: The nursing care for GB syndrome centers on breathing surveillance and offering emotional support. Physical therapy may be used as a rehabilitation strategy. It is essential for patient education on aspects of recovery expectation, potential complications, and follow-up services.

Question: What role does a nurse play while handling traumatic brain injury (TBI)?
Answer: Nurses must continually assess the patient's neurological state, manage complications, and implement rehabilitation techniques for patients with traumatic brain injuries. Daily life support, as well as psychological help, is critical. They educate patients on expected recovery, preventing disease recurrence, and possible approval.

Question: What should the nursing care of a patient with migraine and headache include?
Answer: The assessment of triggers and provision of medications should be done during migraine or headache nursing care. Non-pharmacological therapies like relaxation methods are among them. Recommendations can include lifestyle changes such as stress-management strategies. Patients should be educated about trigger recognition, taking their medications as prescribed, and prevention strategies.

Question: What are the nursing interventions for spinal cord injury?
Answer: Spinal cord injury nursing care includes managing complications, facilitating normal activities, ADLs, and rehabilitation approaches. Working with the health care team for surgical interventions and medications is essential. There is a need for patient education on adaptive techniques, preventive measures as well as existing resources.

Question: What does nursing care entail in terms of managing peripheral neuropathy?
Answer: Patients' self-care should involve pain relieving, making necessary lifestyle changes, and alerting healthcare providers of potential complications. It is essential to work alongside healthcare providers whose tasks should focus on medication adjustment and additional interventions. It is also necessary to educate patients on self-care, symptom management, and the need for routine follow-up.

Question: What is the treatment for neuromuscular disorders in nursing care?
Answer: Symptom management, assistance with ADLs, and collaboration with other health professionals are essential aspects of nursing care regarding neuromuscular disorders. Physical therapy and different rehabilitation strategies. Patient education should be on disease progression, ways they can adapt, and available support services.

Question: What does the management of sleep disorders look like in nursing care?
Answer: Screening on sleeping habits, applying sleep hygienic procedures, and working with doctors on interventions like CPAP treatment is an essential part of nursing care for sleeping disorders. It is crucial for patient education regarding sleep hygiene, lifestyle modification, and follow-up.

Question: Describe managing a patient undergoing acute renal failure.
Answer: A nursing intervention plan entails regular monitoring of fluid balance and electrolytes and medication administration to an AKI patient. Further, a preventive strategy is imperative. Dialysis may be indicated. Patients must receive education on dietary restrictions, fluid management, and postoperative follow-up care.

Question: What does a nurse have as their job when dealing with a patient who has been found after a drug overdose?
Answer: During managing such a patient, the nurse assesses vital signs, administers antidotes/supportive care & monitors for complications. Collaborating with the healthcare team, including the mental health professionals, is essential. Educating patients on the issue of medication safety, overdose prevention, and information access for further research is necessary.

Question: Explain managing a patient with alcohol withdrawal syndrome in nursing care.
Answer: Nursing care entails constant assessment of withdrawal symptoms, giving drugs like benzodiazepines, and emotional support. They may need to team up with addiction specialists. Educating the patient on the dangers of alcohol withdrawal, how one can cope with this problem, and what kind of support is available should be paramount.

Question: The nursing considerations for the patient on blood transfusions.
Answer: Nursing issues encompass checking blood compatibility, monitoring vital signs during the transfusion, and the aftermath of the transfusion reactions. The patient needs to be educated on the process of transfusion and possible adverse reactions, among other things, as well as about unfavorable side effects.

Question: How does a nurse handle a DVT?
Answer: The nursing care for deep vein thrombosis involves the provision of anticoagulants, monitoring complications, and mobilizing patient. The best thing a nurse can do is apply compression and elevate the leg of an affected patient with an ankle injury. Patients must be informed about medication compliance, identification of a second episode, and what precautions to take.

Question: What is the justification for caring for a patient post-heart operation?
Answer: Post-cardiac surgery care includes managing vital signs, relieving pain, preventing complications such as infection or bleeding, and promoting mobility. Likewise, there is a need for respiration care, e.g., breathing exercises. Education of the patient on wound care, medications, and lifestyle changes is required.

Question: What do nurses do for patients who suffered strokes?
Answer: Post-stroke nursing encompasses monitoring vital signs, neuro assessment, and measures to prevent subsequent complications. Physical therapy, speech, and occupational therapy are essential for rehabilitation strategies. They should educate patients about stroke recovery, medication, and living healthy lifestyles.

Question: How is epilepsy managed in nursing care?
Answer: Nursing care is aimed at the administration of antiepileptic drugs, observation of seizure activities, and teaching patients how to handle medical prescriptions and seizure causations. Collaborating with healthcare providers for proper medication adjustments and frequent follow-ups is imperative. Such patient education should include lifestyle modification and recognition of early warning signs.

Question: What role does nursing care have in managing neurodegenerative disease?
Answer: The management of symptoms, assistance with activities of daily living, and monitoring for complications are hallmarks of nursing care for neurodegenerative diseases. It is, therefore, imperative that one collaborates with a multidisciplinary healthcare team for medicines and intervention. Educating patients about disease progression, self-management tips, and relevant resources is vital.

Question: In this case, what does a nurse do if a patient's oxygen saturation begins falling off?
Answer: When a patient's oxygen saturation falls, the nurse discovers the cause, provides supplementary oxygen, and keeps track of the respiratory status carefully. Such prompt interventions may involve increasing or reducing the oxygen flow rate, repositioning the patient towards better ventilation, and applying the healthcare team in further evaluations and interventions.

Question: What is the nursing of a fracture patient, and how are they managed in terms of pain control?
Answer: Evaluating pain intensity, giving analgesia, and checking for adverse effects constitute post-fracture pain management. Such non-pharmacological interventions can include positioning and applying ice may be employed. Education of patients on medication adherence, activity modification, and possible complications is critical.

Question: What specific dieting recommendations are administered to a person who has cirrhosis of the liver?
Answer: Patients having liver cirrhosis should be advised on a low sodium diet, minimization of consumption of alcohol, and checking protein intake. This diet should consist of small but regular meals which contain as many vitamins and minerals as possible. The patient must have a proper orientation concerning fluid balance, nutritional options, and the necessity of follow-up visits.

Question: What do you do for a patient who avoids asthma attacks?
Answer: Asthmatic attacks can be prevented by identifying triggers, adhering to medication, and designing an asthma action plan. These include long-term control medication such as inhaled corticosteroids and bronchodilators. Patients must learn to identify early symptoms, use an inhaler correctly, and visit a doctor promptly.

Question: What is involved in caring for a patient with thyroid disorder?
Answer: Nursing interventions during thyroid problems include administering medicines, monitoring TFT, and observing for possible complications. Effective patient management includes education about compliance with medications, dietary considerations, and the need for routine follow-ups.

Question: How is MS treated in nursing care?
Answer: For nursing care of MS, there are disease-modifying drugs to be administered, followed by symptom management and emotional support. Such strategies for rehabilitating patients may include physical and occupational therapy. Patient education regarding medication adherence, symptom management, and healthy lifestyle changes is critical.

Question: What management strategies does a nurse use for a patient with amyotrophic lateral sclerosis?
Answer: Therefore, nurse care for ALS includes helping with activities of daily living, symptom management, and collaboration with healthcare providers for medical interventions. These include palliative care and emotional support. The importance of patient education on the nature of the disease, how one adapts, and available support services should be emphasized.

Question: How is the nursing care treatment planned for Guillain-Barre Syndrome?
Answer: Supportive nursing care, with administering immunoglobulins or plasmapheresis, is required concerning the respiratory functions of a patient suffering from this syndrome. Physical therapy may also be initiated as part of rehabilitation strategies. Patients' knowledge about recovery expectations, possible complications, and post-patient care is critical.

Question: What is TBI management in nursing care?
Care in nursing for TBI requires monitoring neurological status, treating complications, and rehabilitation measures. This kind of supportive care includes supporting activities of daily living and emotional well-being. Therefore, it is essential to educate patients on their recovery expectations, precautionary practices, and available resources to facilitate treatment.

Question: Describe the Management of migraine or headache by nursing.
Answer: In nursing of migraine and headache, there is evaluation of triggers, administration of drugs, and non-pharmacologic measures such as relaxation. This can include lifestyle changes or stress control. It is essential for patient education on identifying triggers, ensuring medication compliance, and preventive measures.

Question: What is involved in dealing with a patient with a broken bone?
Answer: When taking care of a person who has a fractured bone, it is necessary to prevent movements, manage pain, and pay attention to possible further complications. Educating the patient about cast change, activity restrictions, and the importance of future visits is essential.

Question: Explain the management of sprains and strains in nursing care.
Answer: Sprain and strain nursing care entails the RICE approach and pain management. It is essential to give education about self-care measures, activity modification, and graduated return to normal activities.

Question: What are the procedures for caring for osteoarthritis (OA)?
Answer: The nursing care for OA comprises pain therapy, joint care, and lifestyle change. Partners of healthcare providers in prescription and rehab interventions are required. It includes patient education about symptom management and joint-friendly activities.

Question: How should you go about treating the RA in your care facility?
Answer: RA nursing care entails the prescription of DMARDS, alleviating symptoms, and enhancing knee articulation. Making changes in the medication and its close monitoring with the health care team is very important. A patient must be educated on medication adherence, joint protection, and any necessary lifestyle modification.

Question: What do the nurses do when managing osteoporosis in those they are caring for?
Answer: Calcium and vitamin- D supplementations are used in nursing care for osteoporosis, while drugs that increase bone density also are used in nursing care. In addition, fall prevention strategies are used in nursing care for osteoporosis. Working with specialists like pediatricians, obstetricians-gynecologists, and psychiatrists for prevention means and control is necessary. It is imperative for patient education on bone issues, falls, and lifestyle modifications.

Question: How does a nurse deal with musculoskeletal back pain in a patient?
Answer: Pain relief and education on good body mechanics with exercise for strength and flexibility constitute nursing care for musculoskeletal back pain. Shared imaging and intervention with healthcare providers are paramount. Such patient education involves back care, posture, and preventive measures.

Question: Can intervention be utilized for controlling gout among nurses?
Answer: When it comes to nursing care for gout, analgesia is applied, as well as reducing the level of uric acid in the blood and food modifications. This intervention has three main aspects—education on trigger foods, medicine compliance, and lifestyle changes.

Question: How does fibromyalgia impact nursing care?
Answer: Fibromyalgia requires pain management, good sleep habits, and light workouts while receiving nurses' care. Health care provider collaboration should provide medications, and psychosocial support should include education on self-care measures, reduction of stress levels, and lifestyle modification.

Question: What is the best way for a nurse to manage SLE?
Answer: Nursing care for SLE includes the management of symptoms, the provision of appropriate medication such as corticosteroids, and the provision of counseling. Collaborating with the clinicians on follow-up is essential for monitoring the disease progression and interventions. It is necessary for a health professional to teach medication adherence, symptom identification, and dietary modification in patients.

Question: What is Tendinitis management for a nurse on a patient?
Answer: The treatment for tendinitis involves pain relief, rest, and the application of ice and some warmth, depending on the swelling condition. The healthcare providers should be working together with medication and rehabilitation interventions. The nurse should educate patients, modify their activity, proper warm-ups, and preventive options.

Question: Explain Nursing management of carpal tunnel syndrome.
Answer: Splinting, analgesia, and fitting the patient with appropriate equipment are some treatments for carpal tunnel syndrome. Working with healthcare providers for surgical interventions and corticosteroid injections is critical. It requires educating patients on wrist protection, activity modifications, and prevention measures.

Question: Describe Musculoskeletal nursing care interventions in pain management.
Answer: Pain management for MSN care entails assessment of pain, giving analgesics, and applying cold or heat. The client should work hand in hand with the health care team as they always carry out continuous monitoring and pain control. However, it is equally crucial to teach patients about pain management methods and side effects that may arise.

Question: What is the significance of musculoskeletal nursing physiotherapy/ rehabilitation?
Answer: Exercise programs designed to enhance movement and stimulate recovery in musculoskeletal nursing care in physical therapies and rehabilitation. It entails collaborating with physiologists and healthcare providers to develop personalized regimes. Patients must be informed about adherence to exercise therapeutic objectives and that there is no reason to miss a therapy session.

Question: What is the role of orthotic devices in musculoskeletal nursing practice?
Answer: Musculoskeletal muscular nursing care refers to evaluating and fitting orthotic equipment on the patients, including braces, splints, and support apparatuses. Regular monitoring with the collaboration of orthopedic specialists is needed for individual device adjustment. Therefore, patient education on appropriate usage, maintenance, and possible alterations will be crucial.

Question: What surgeries do you utilize in your musculoskeletal nursing care regimen?
Answer: Musculoskeletal nursing care interventions may include surgical treatments like joint replacement, fracture fixation, and spinal surgery. Nursing care includes preoperative preparation, postoperative monitoring, and working with the surgeons. It is essential for patient education in post-surgery care, rehabilitation, and restricting activities.

Question: Explain Incorporating lifestyle modifications into musculoskeletal nursing care.
Answer: Musculoskeletal lifestyle alterations include healthy practices, weight control, and the modification of an active schedule that lessens the burden on joints. It's essential to work together with healthcare practitioners for individualized strategies. Education of patients on the need for lifestyle change is crucial for good symptom management and general health.

Question: What is the role of supplementary therapies (musculoskeletal nursing)?
Answer: In musculoskeletal nursing care, these approaches include, among other things, acupuncture, massage, and herbal medicines. Healthcare providers and complementary therapy specialists must work together. The patient's education on complementary therapies' probable outcomes and disadvantages must be addressed.

Question: What approaches are applied in medication management under muscular nursing care?
Answer: Musculoskeletal nursing care encompasses the prescription of medication, monitoring for adverse reactions, and collaboration with physicians on dose adjustment. Education of patients about medicine adherence, possible side effects, and the need for periodic checking is paramount.

Question: Psychosocial support and its significance in musculoskeletal nursing care.
Answer: Musculoskeletal nursing psychosocial support encompasses providing for the emotional and mental health of those with chronic disorders. Working together with psychiatrists and patient groups is inevitable. Educating patients about coping strategies, mental health resources, and available support services is essential.

Question: What is intravenous and subcutaneous therapy's role in musculoskeletal care?
Answer: Musculoskeletal nursing care includes intravenous and subcutaneous therapies, which mean giving an injection for various diseases involving the bones, such as rheumatoid arthritis and osteoporosis. Working hand-in-hand with healthcare professionals responsible for proper dosing and surveillance is essential. Therefore, patient education regarding the need for regular treatments and possible adverse reactions and information on future care is also crucial.

Question: What happens if you have a hyperextension and someone puts pressure on it?
Answer: Dietary changes, exercise, and drug compliance as measures of hypertension management. For blood pressure not to exceed a specific limit, hypertension is treated by using different drugs like ace inhibitors and beta blockers. Care involves periodic blood pressure measurements and patient education on self-care and management programs.

Question: What are some post-operational care services offered to a patient?
Answer: Post-cardiac surgery care includes vital signs monitoring, pain management, bleed prevention, and reduction, as well as promotion of mobility. Respiratory care is dependent on deep breathing exercises. This entails educating patients on wound care, drug administration, and lifestyle modifications for adequate healing.

Question: For stroke and in the caring of a patient, what is essential?
Answer: Stroke care involves rapid assessment of stroke mechanisms, risk factors, and protective interventions against brain degeneration. The monitoring of vital signs, treating complications involving dysphagia, and engaging in rehabilitative strategies. In the long run, management demands being aware of preventive measures, medication, and lifestyle changes.

Question: What is the management of diabetes by a patient?
Answer: Regularly checking the blood sugar, taking the medication as advised, and eating balanced and healthy diets with enough exercise are all part of managing or controlling diabetes. It might involve instructing dietary measures, prescribing insulin, or oral hypoglycemic agents. Effective diabetes management involves enlightening patients on symptoms, complications, and self-care.

Question: Do nurses control pressure ulcers appropriately?
Answer: It consists of continuous examination, taking it easy, and maintaining wound hygiene. This is one of the critical areas that includes dressing changes, infection control, and nutritional support. Prevention also comprises key elements like skin care, repositioning, and moisture control as essential management.

Question: What nursing care is given to a patient with kidney disease?
Answer: The nursing care for kidney patients includes monitoring fluid and electrolyte balance, administering medication for blood pressure and related symptoms, and restricting specific diets. Patients must be able to educate themselves on proper management of medicine, necessary and healthy diet changes, and timely check-ups.

Question: Why should you not consider chemotherapy for a cancer patient?
Answer: Some of chemotherapy's complications are nausea, tiredness, immunosuppression, and toxicity of organs. This includes monitoring for adverse effects, giving supportive treatments, and offering emotional support. This is important in patient education regarding possible side effects, self-care activities, and follow-up visits.

Question: What is done for the management of burns in a patient?
Answer: Burn management comprises wound assessment, pain control, and prevention of the infection process. Critical elements of care include dressing's changes, fluid resuscitation, and nutritional support. Good outcome toward recovery involves educating patients about wound management, scar prevention, and the importance of follow-up appointments.

Question: How are COPD patients managed in nursing care?
Answer: The treatment of COPD includes bronchodilators and oxygen therapy, as well as implementing measures to enhance respiratory function. Respiratory monitoring, medication administration, and inhaler instruction with symptom management are aspects of nursing care.

Question: How would you go about taking care of a patient suffering from heart failure?
Answer: Patients with HF should adhere well to their medications and monitor fluids (intake); signs of HF aggravation must be checked out. Specific lifestyle modifications like limiting salt intake and exercising regularly are essential. This involves educating patients on symptom recognition, medication management, and appointment compliance.

Question: What do you need to know when handling a patient with a neurological illness such as Parkinson's disease?
Answer: Medication administration, symptom monitoring (both motor and non-motor), and assistance in movement are components of nursing care for a patient with Parkinson's syndrome. Such supportive therapies as physical and occupational therapy are also vital. The patient's education on medication schedules, safety, and self-care at home is critical.

Question: How does the nurse assist patients with sepsis?
Answer: Early identification by the nurse, early administration of antibiotics, and maintenance of hemodynamic stability are essential for sepsis management. Tracking vitals, administering fluids, and cooperating with the nursing staff are crucial factors. This type of patient education focuses on teaching patients how to prevent infections, recognize early signs, and seek immediate medical care for illnesses.

Question: What is done to prepare the patient to undergo the surgery?
Answer: The process of preparing a patient for surgery includes getting informed consent per the HEC code of conduct and preoperative screening followed by preoperative education. The fasting is properly ensured, pre-anesthesia medications are issued, and the patient's concerns are addressed. Education of a patient regarding postoperative care, recovery expectancy, and subsequent appointments is a must.

Question: How should a nurse plan to care for patients going through radiotherapy?
Answer: Nursing considerations include proper skin care, managing symptoms, and counseling the patient undergoing radiotherapy. The health professional should monitor side effects, teach the patient essential safety measures, and work with other team members in radiation oncology. Patient education about possible complications, self-care measures, and appointments for follow-up is of utmost importance.

Question: What should a nurse do to maintain a pneumonia patient?
Answer: Administration of antibiotics, assessment of respiratory status, and hydration are integral parts of nursing care for a patient with pneumonia. Chest physiotherapy and breathing exercises can be used to promote better lung functions. Patients need to know how to stick to medication plans, recognize symptoms, and not stop treatment prematurely.

Question: What is incorporated in nursing practice for wound care?
Answer: In the nursing practice, wound care involves assessment, cleansing, dressings, and observing indications of infections. Suggested strategies could include advanced therapies like, for example, negative pressure wound therapy. Patients need to be educated about self-monitoring, wound protection, and post-appointment.

Question: What can a nurse do for a suffering patient?
Answer: When treating patients with pain, their pain level is ascertained before a decision on medication is made, and after that, their response is monitored to prevent any adverse side effects. This includes positioning as well as some non-medical strategies for relaxation. Patients must be informed about pain control strategies, medication compliance, and possible complications.

Question: What educational methods are used for patients during nursing practice?
Answer: Assessment of patients' learning needs, informing clearly, and applying different teaching strategies are part of patient education in nursing practice. These include written texts, demonstrations, and oral communication. Education of a patient involves issues on self-care, administering medication, and lifestyle changes.

Question: What is the healthcare provider's role in controlling diabetes in patients?
Answer: The four pillars of diabetes management are blood glucose control, medication adherence, healthy diet, and physical activity. Doctors may advise on insulin or an oral hypoglycemic compound—patient education on self-care for diabetes symptoms and complications.

Question: How are pressure ulcers managed in nursing care?
Answer: Periodic assessment, offloading pressure to the affected area, and wound cleaning are part of a pressure ulcer care plan. These involve dressing changes, infection control, and nutritional support. It is, therefore, vital that prevention and management of pressure ulcers be explained to the patients on how they should care for their skin, the need to change positions frequently, and the effects of moisture control.

Question: What would a nurse do if oxygen saturation for a patient deteriorates?
Answer: A nurse assesses and determines reasons for a fall in oxygen concentration and provides O2 from a mask with continuous respiratory check-ups. Some immediate steps include changing the oxygen flow rates, repositioning the patient for maximum ventilation, and calling the medical team.

Question: Describe the Patient on the management of burns.
Answer: Burn care involves wound assessment, pain relief, and infection control. For instance, it consists of dressing changes and providing infusion fluids using a pump and feeding. The care of patients for optimal recovery consists of educating them on wound care, scar prevention, and post-care follow-ups.

Question: What is the nurse's role in managing AKI?
Answer: In caring for an AKI patient, determining causes is important, together with managing fluid and electrolytes and avoiding complications. These include monitoring renal function, use of medication administration, and giving nutrition advice.

CONCLUSION

As we draw this comprehensive guide to a close, let's revisit the journey we've embarked on. Throughout this text, we've explored the vast domain of Medical-Surgical Nursing, delved into the complexities of specialized areas, dissected the intricacies of patient care, and addressed the professional issues every nurse encounters.

This endeavor aimed to serve as a guide and a companion for nurses venturing into medical-surgical nursing. We've uncovered the essence of this multidimensional field by exploring the distinct sections of Cardiovascular, Pulmonary, Gastrointestinal, Renal, Urinary, Neurological, Musculoskeletal, Endocrine, and Hematological and Immunological Nursing. We've navigated disease processes, interventions, treatments, and patient management strategies through each section.

The depth of knowledge required in these areas is significant, given the variety of conditions patients may present with. Therefore, we aimed to provide a baseline understanding and a roadmap for further exploration and professional development in each nursing field.

Simultaneously, we acknowledged the crucial role of ethical principles, legal responsibilities, and evidence-based practices in nursing. Our discussions on these subjects illuminated the importance of adhering to the highest standards of patient care, advocacy, and ongoing education.

In patient safety and quality improvement, we outlined methodologies for nurses to cultivate an environment that prioritizes patient well-being and reduces risks. We explored the necessity of a safety culture in healthcare settings and nurses' role in building this culture.

As we worked our way through practice questions and FAQs about the CMSRN exam, we provided you with tools to gauge your understanding and readiness. These questions, designed to be challenging yet comprehensive, mirrored the complexity of real-world scenarios, stimulating critical thinking and problem-solving skills.

Our journey ends here, but your professional voyage continues. This book is not an endpoint, but a stepping-stone, fueling your curiosity, expanding your knowledge, and enhancing your skills. We sincerely hope that the information, insights, and resources presented in this book empower you to strive for excellence in your nursing practice, improve patient outcomes, and achieve professional fulfilment.
The world of medical-surgical nursing, as are the challenges and rewards it presents, is ever-evolving. May this book be a beacon that guides you along the path of continual learning, inspiring you to dive deeper, reach higher, and grow further in your nursing career?

SPECIAL EXTRA CONTENT

Congratulations on Completing This Educational Journey!

Dear esteemed reader, If these final words are resonating with you, it signifies that you have successfully navigated through a path of personal and professional development, and we are privileged to have been part of your journey towards knowledge.

Your Insights Are Invaluable!

Your experiences, reflections, and feedback on the material you've just completed are crucial to us. We earnestly encourage you to share your thoughts about our book on Amazon. Whether a particular section struck a chord with you or the overall journey through the pages has broadened your understanding, your perspective is immensely important. By sharing your experiences, you help guide other learners and provide us, the authors, with the inspiration needed to refine our work and continue delivering impactful content.

Uncover Special EXTRA CONTENT Reserved Just for You!

In appreciation of your commitment, we've prepared exclusive additional content specifically for our readers. Here's what awaits you:

- *Audiobook* ready to rock on your drive, at the gym, wherever you choose!
- **eBook** titled *"Medical Terminology for Health Careers"*
- **+ 600 Flashcards <u>WITH PICTUREs</u>** of *"Medical Terms"* for easier recall and understanding.
  Note. FLASHCARDS ARE READY TO USE FOR FREE online or offline! You can track your progress and conveniently and interactively memorize the most important terms and concepts! Download to your device: Anki APP or Anki Droid, or enter the web page and register free of charge. Then import the files we have given you as a gift and use the flashcards whenever and wherever you want to study and track your progress.
- Broad-ranging **case studies** on various aspects of medical-surgical nursing, including the *management of chronic conditions such as diabetes* and *rheumatoid arthritis, clinical communication, patient safety, ethics, pain management,* and *care in diverse settings like the ICU and pediatric ward.*

Straightforward Resources for Ongoing Enrichment

Below, you will find a distinctive QR CODE leading directly to your bonus content, ready for immediate download and exploration. There's no need for email subscriptions or personal detail disclosures; this is our direct gift to you, supporting your continued educational journey seamlessly.

Should you encounter any issues or have any questions regarding the downloadable material, please feel free to reach out to us at **booklovers.1001@gmail.com**

Sending warm regards and best wishes for your future endeavors.
With heartfelt thanks!
We look forward to your feedback!
Thank you!

Made in United States
North Haven, CT
06 July 2024